MW01519411

# the CSIRO
## total wellbeing diet
## recipes on a budget

**The Commonwealth Scientific and Industrial Research Organisation (CSIRO)**, Australia's national science agency, has been dedicated to the practical application of knowledge and science for society and industry since 1928. Today the CSIRO ranks in the top one per cent of world scientific institutions in twelve out of twenty-two research fields. CSIRO Animal, Food and Health Sciences conducts research into human health, including disease prevention, diagnosis and innovative treatment.

**Professor Manny Noakes** is the Research Program Leader for CSIRO Animal, Food and Health Sciences. With her team, she conducts research that provides scientific evidence for the efficacy of diet and exercise programs on health. Manny has published over one hundred scientific papers, with a major emphasis on diet composition, weight-loss and cardiovascular health.

csiro.au

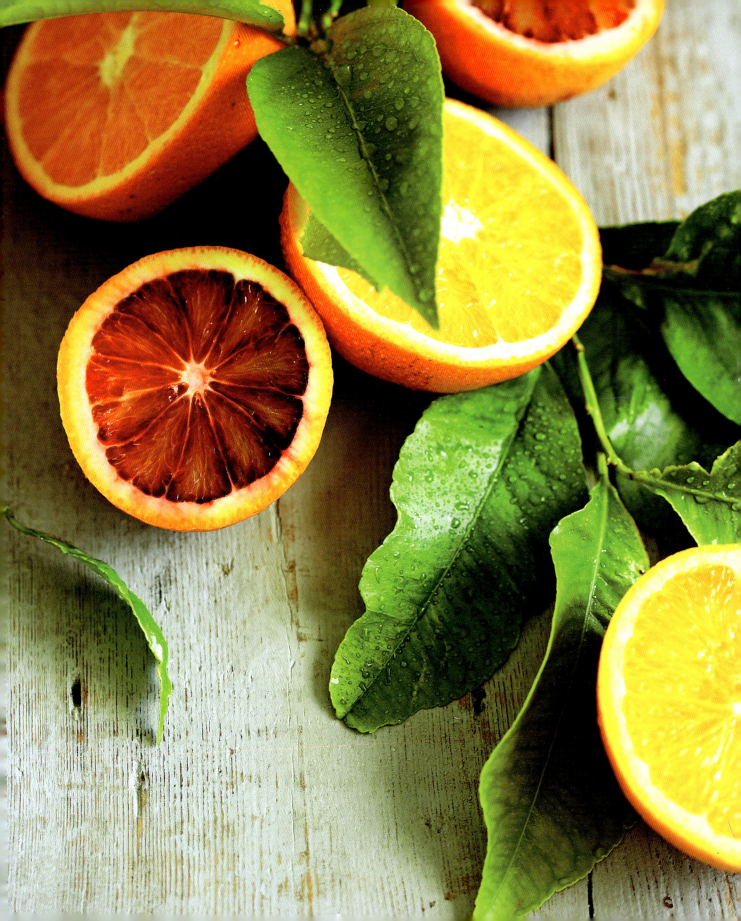

# the CSIRO
# total wellbeing diet
# recipes on a budget

**Introduction by Dr Manny Noakes**  Photography by Cath Muscat

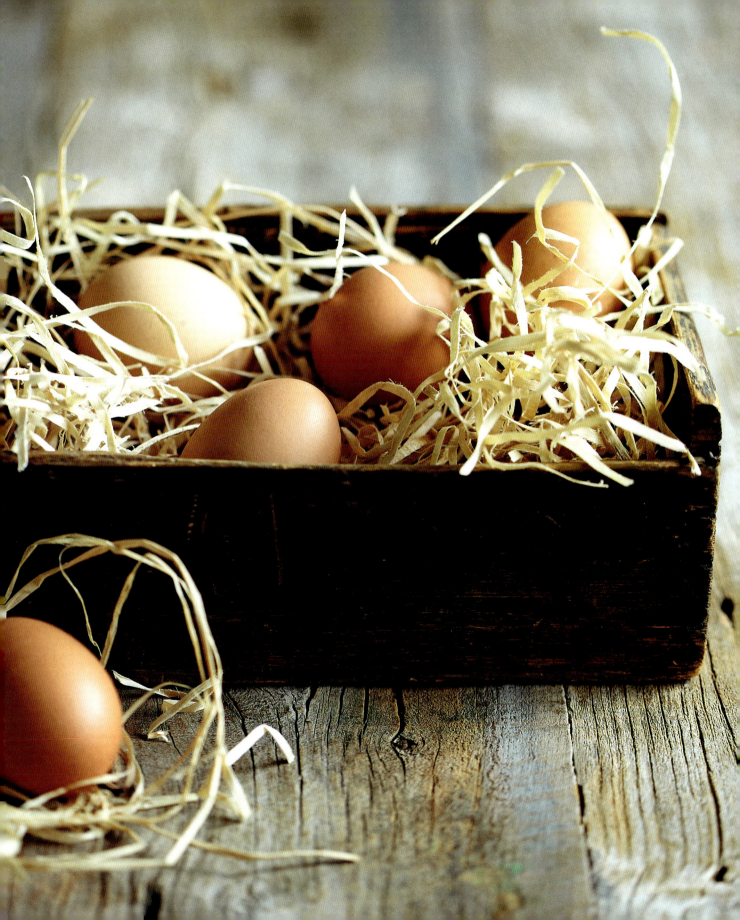

# contents

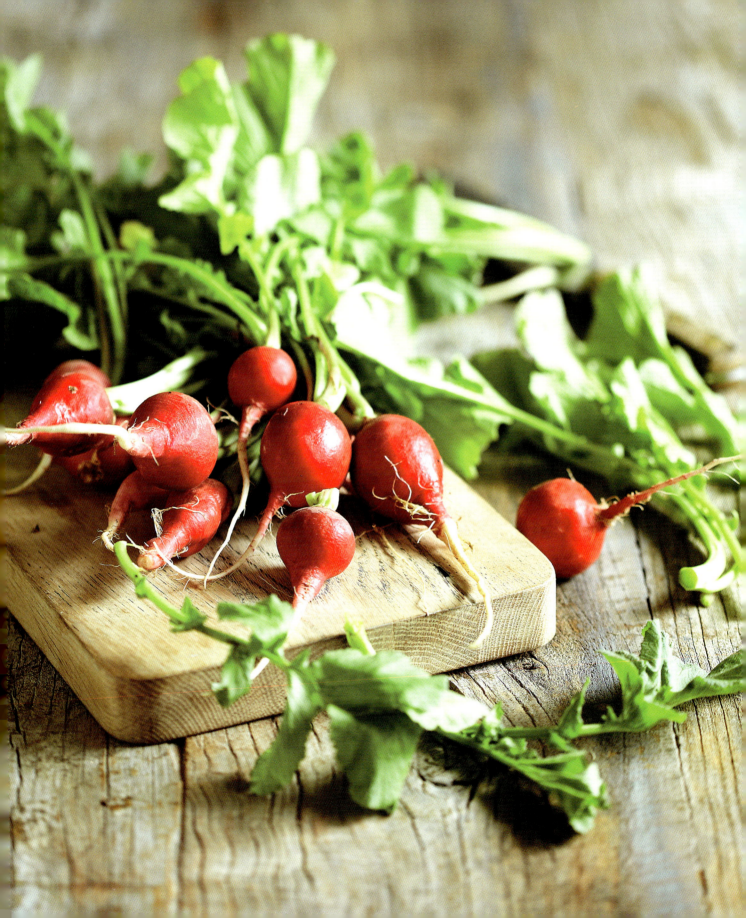

# introduction

These days, watching what we spend on food has become a necessity for many of us. Here at CSIRO, we know that it can sometimes be difficult to stick to a budget while eating for good health, so this new recipe book helps you to do both. Packed full of ideas and tips, it's devoted to those of us who want to economise on food without compromising on flavour or nutrition.

The Total Wellbeing Diet includes ingredients from all food groups, so there's no need to miss out on anything, and the recipes are designed to use everyday items in your pantry. We begin with some clever ideas for recreating healthy, low-cost versions of those delicious cafe-style breakfasts and brunches. There's a section on vegetables, salads and soups that will ensure you get your five serves a day, and there are sweet treats too: delicious puddings, muffins and fruit dishes that draw on the dairy, fruit and grain food groups. When it comes to buying fruit and vegetables, remember that what's in season will always be cheaper – and it will taste better too.

We've included a chapter devoted to slow-cooked recipes. Slow cooking is perfect for transforming budget cuts of meat into hearty meals without affecting any of the essential minerals they contain. There is a great collection of chicken and fish recipes too, as well as some tasty and exciting vegetarian meals.

So often we use salt as the main way to flavour our meals, yet too much salt can increase blood pressure and cause deterioration of our blood vessel walls. Using herbs and spices to enhance flavour is a much healthier option, and there are plenty of ideas on how to do this here. Spices are cheap to buy, can be stored over a relatively long period and a little bit goes a long way. Simple guidelines on growing your own herbs will bring out your inner gardener, and the fruits of your labour can be used in myriad ways. As the cost of buying fresh herbs can really add up, this is a perfect way to have a ready supply. Talking about adding flavour, check out the Basics section, too, which includes recipes for delicious dips, pastes, dressings and spice mixes that are inexpensive to make but really add pizazz to your cooking.

Minimising food waste is good for your budget (and good for the planet as well), so with this in mind we've included a section on how to use leftovers to make substantial meals. With a bit of forward planning, this will save you time and money in the long run, and you'll be amazed at the delicious meals you can create second time around.

We hope you enjoy this latest collection of Total Wellbeing Diet recipes, and have fun expanding your repertoire of recipes for all occasions.

Dr Manny Noakes

# the CSIRO total wellbeing diet
## basic plan

## Your daily food allowance

### LEAN PROTEIN FOODS
**– 2 units a day for dinner**

1 unit is equal to 100 g raw weight of protein food, including red meat, chicken or fish (without bones). Eat red meat 3 times a week for dinner. Eat fish at least twice a week for dinner.

**– up to 1 unit a day for lunch**

Eat up to 100 g (raw weight) of any lean protein source (tinned or fresh fish or seafood, chicken, turkey, red meat or 2 eggs) each day for lunch. Eat red meat up to once a week for lunch.

### WHOLEGRAIN BREAD
**– 2 units a day**

1 unit is equal to one 35 g slice. You can replace 1 unit each day with any of the following:
- 1 slice fruit loaf
- 2 crispbread, such as Ryvita
- 1 medium potato (about 150 g)
- 4 tablespoons cooked rice or noodles
- ½ cup (about 50 g) cooked pasta
- 4 tablespoons baked beans, or cooked lentils, kidney beans or other legumes
- 40 g high-fibre cereal or rolled oats

### HIGH-FIBRE CEREAL
**– 1 unit a day**

1 unit is equal to:
- 40 g any high-fibre breakfast cereal (e.g. Sultana Bran, Fibre Plus)
- 1 Weet-Bix plus ½ cup (35 g) All-Bran
- 40 g rolled oats
- 1 slice wholegrain toast

### DAIRY
**– 3 units a day**

1 unit is equal to:
- 250 ml reduced-fat milk
- 200 g reduced-fat or diet yoghurt
- 200 g reduced-fat custard or dairy dessert
- 25 g cheddar cheese or other full-fat cheese
- 50 g reduced-fat cheese (less than 10 per cent fat)

### FRUIT
**– 2 units a day**

1 unit is equal to 150 g fresh or tinned unsweetened fruit, 150 ml unsweetened fruit juice or 30 g dried fruit.

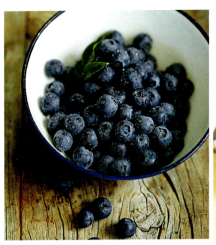
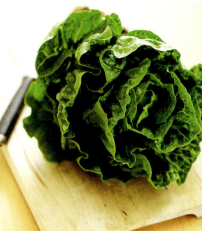
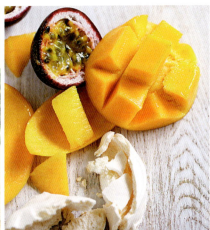

## VEGETABLES
**– at least 2½ units a day from free list**

1 unit is equal to 1 cup (80–150 g) cooked vegetables. See free list (right) for vegetables you can eat. We recommend ½ unit salad and 2 cups (160–300 g) cooked vegetables each day.

## FATS AND OILS
**– 3 units added oils or fats a day**

1 unit is equal to 1 teaspoon any liquid oil such as canola, olive or sunflower oil. 3 units oil is equal to:
• 3 teaspoons soft (trans-fat-free) margarine
• 6 teaspoons light margarine
• 3 teaspoons curry paste in canola oil
• 60 g avocado
• 20 g nuts or seeds

## INDULGENCE FOODS
**– up to 2 units a week**

This depends on the level of plan best for you (see *The CSIRO Total Wellbeing Diet* books 1 and 2). As a general rule, 1 unit is equal to any food or drink providing approximately 450 kJ, such as 150 ml wine or 20 g chocolate.

## THE FREE LIST: ANYTIME FOODS

The vegetables below contain minimal kilojoules, so eat them freely with your meals.

Artichokes, asparagus, bamboo shoots, bean sprouts, beetroot, bok choy, broccoli, broccolini, brussels sprouts, cabbage, capsicum, carrots, cauliflower, celeriac, celery, chilli, Chinese broccoli, chives, choko, choy sum, corn, cucumber, eggplant, fennel, fresh herbs, green beans, kohlrabi, leeks, lettuce, marrow, mushrooms, onion, parsnips, peas, pumpkin, radishes, rhubarb, rocket, silverbeet, snowpeas, spinach, swedes, tomatoes, turnip, zucchini.

## READING THE RECIPES IN THIS BOOK

The nutritional units contained in each recipe are displayed above the recipe.

## FOR MORE INFORMATION

Please refer to *The CSIRO Total Wellbeing Diet* books 1 and 2 for more extensive diet and lifestyle information.

# sample weekly meal plan

|  | MONDAY | TUESDAY | WEDNESDAY |
|---|---|---|---|
| **BREAKFAST** | **Breakfast smoothies** (pg 12) | Pear, strawberry and kiwifruit bircher muesli (pg 14) topped with a sprinkle of slivered almonds | 200 g reduced-fat or diet yoghurt, topped with 20 g high-fibre cereal, 1 grated apple, 20 g crushed nuts and sprinkled with cinnamon (optional) |
|  | ½ unit cereal<br>1 unit dairy<br>1 unit fruit | 1 unit cereal<br>½ unit dairy<br>½ unit fruit<br>1 unit fats | ½ unit cereal<br>1 unit dairy<br>1 unit fruit<br>1 unit fats |
| **LUNCH** | **Tuna salad cups with paprika crisps** (pg 42) plus 200 g reduced-fat or diet yoghurt OR 200 g reduced-fat custard | **Ginger-steamed tofu with stir-fried vegetables** (pg 52) served with 50 g cooked basmati rice plus 200 g reduced-fat or diet yoghurt | **Indian-spiced chicken wrap** (pg 139) plus 150 ml unsweetened fruit juice and 150 g diet dairy dessert |
|  | 1 unit protein<br>1 unit bread<br>1 unit dairy<br>2 units vegetables<br>1 unit fats | 1 unit protein<br>1 unit bread<br>1 unit dairy<br>2 units vegetables<br>1 unit fats | 1 unit protein<br>1 unit bread<br>1 unit dairy<br>1 unit fruit<br>1½ units vegetables |
| **DINNER** | **Middle Eastern shepherd's pie with pumpkin and green beans** (pg 71) plus 1 x 40 g multigrain roll and 5 g monounsaturated-fat margarine<br><br>Supper: 1 small skim latte plus 4 strawberries | **Indian-spiced roast chicken with warm carrot and radish salad** (pg 102)<br><br>Supper: **Spiced ricotta fruit toast** (pg 16) | **Chicken baked in a bread crust with lentil salad** (pg 110) plus 50 g reduced-fat feta and 10 g avocado (sliced and tossed through the salad) |
|  | 2 units protein<br>1½ units bread<br>1 unit dairy<br>1 unit fruit<br>3 units vegetables<br>2 units fats | 2 units protein<br>1 unit bread<br>½ unit dairy<br>½ unit fruit<br>2 units vegetables<br>1 unit fats | 2 units protein<br>1½ units bread<br>1 unit dairy<br>1½ units vegetables<br>2 units fats |
| **DAILY SNACKS** | No snack required | 1 piece of fresh fruit plus 1 small skim latte | No snack required |
|  |  | 1 unit dairy<br>1 unit fruit |  |

| THURSDAY | FRIDAY | SATURDAY | SUNDAY |
|---|---|---|---|
| Pear, strawberry and kiwifruit bircher muesli (pg 14) topped with a sprinkle of slivered almonds | 200 g reduced-fat or diet yoghurt topped with 40 g high-fibre cereal, a thinly sliced banana and a drizzle of honey | 200 g reduced-fat or diet vanilla yoghurt topped with 40 g high-fibre cereal and 150 g mixed berries | Brunch: **Soft-boiled eggs with cheesy soldiers and baked mushrooms** (pg 20) plus 1 cup (250 ml) skim milk or 200 g reduced-fat or diet yoghurt |
| 1 unit cereal<br>½ unit dairy<br>½ unit fruit<br>1 unit fats | 1 unit cereal<br>1 unit dairy<br>1 unit fruit | 1 unit bread<br>1 unit dairy<br>1 unit fruit | |
| Deluxe chicken sandwich (pg 137) plus 1 piece of fresh fruit OR 150 g fresh fruit salad | 100 g tinned tuna or salmon, 1 cup (40 g) mixed greens, ½ grated carrot and 50 g grated reduced-fat cheese topped with 1 serve of **Garlic Yoghurt Dressing** (pg 207) wrapped in 1 piece of wholemeal pita | Creamy chicken and mushroom soup with rocket pesto (pg 40) sprinkled with 15 g grated parmesan plus 4 rye Cruskits topped with ½ a thinly sliced tomato or cucumber and cracked pepper | |
| 1 unit protein<br>2 units bread<br>1 unit fruit<br>1 unit vegetables<br>1 unit fats | 1 unit protein<br>1 unit bread<br>1 unit dairy<br>1½ units vegetables<br>1 unit fats | 1 unit protein<br>1½ units bread<br>½ unit dairy<br>2 units vegetables<br>1½ units fats | 1 unit protein<br>1 unit bread<br>2 units dairy<br>1 unit vegetables<br>½ unit fats |
| Simple Thai green fish curry (pg 90) served with a tossed green salad plus 1 serve **Pickled Vegetables** (pg 201) and 25 g reduced-fat cheddar cheese<br>Supper: **Eton mess with passionfruit and mango** (pg 188) | Oregano and lemon chicken with Greek salad (pg 121) served with **Braised red cabbage with honey and mustard** (pg 150)<br>Supper: **1 frozen yoghurt pop** (pg 176) | Thai-style san choi bao (pg 92)<br>Supper: **Apple and watermelon jelly with lemon-lime granita** (pg 187) topped with 150 g reduced-fat or diet vanilla yoghurt | Roast beef with beetroot, onions and chimichurri salsa (pg 74) plus 150 ml unsweetened fruit juice and 1 medium baked potato<br>Supper: **Spiced pear and date strudel** (pg 178) topped with 2 tablespoons reduced-fat custard |
| 2 units protein<br>1½ units dairy<br>½ unit fruit<br>3 units vegetables<br>1 unit fats | 2 units protein<br>1 unit bread<br>1 unit dairy<br>½ unit fruit<br>3 units vegetables<br>2 units fats | 2 units protein<br>1 unit dairy<br>1 unit fruit<br>2 units vegetables<br>1 unit fats | 2 units protein<br>1½ units bread<br>1 unit dairy<br>2 units fruit<br>1½ units vegetables<br>2 units fats |
| 200 g reduced-fat or diet yoghurt OR 1 diet dairy dessert | 75 g fresh fruit salad | 1 serve **Apple and cinnamon mini muffins** (pg 190) heated and served with 100 g reduced-fat custard OR 100 g diet dairy dessert | 1 rye Cruskit topped with 10 g avocado and 2 slices each of tomato and cucumber |
| 1 unit dairy | ½ unit fruit | ½ unit dairy<br>½ unit bread | ½ unit bread<br>½ unit vegetables<br>½ unit fats |

# stocking your kitchen on a budget

## IN THE FRIDGE OR FREEZER

- budget cuts of meat, such as beef shin, chuck steak, gravy beef, lamb or pork shoulder, lamb shanks and chicken thighs
- cheeses, such as reduced-fat cheddar, reduced-fat feta and reduced-fat ricotta
- eggs
- filo pastry
- fresh fruit and vegetables, particularly those in season
- fresh herbs (or grow your own)
- frozen vegetables, such as broad beans and peas
- light margarine
- minced beef, chicken or pork
- poultry
- reduced-fat cottage cheese
- reduced-fat cream cheese
- reduced-fat milk
- reduced-fat sour cream
- reduced-fat flavoured, natural or Greek-style yoghurt
- seafood, such as prawns, white fish fillets and mussels
- tofu

## IN THE PANTRY

- baking powder
- breadcrumbs
- breads, such as wholemeal sourdough, tortillas and wraps
- Chinese Shaohsing rice wine
- cornflour
- crispbread
- dried fruit, such as apples, apricots, cranberries and sultanas
- dried herbs
- dried pasta, such as penne, spaghetti and lasagne sheets; try wholegrain varieties
- dried yeast
- flour, such as wholemeal and white plain flours
- grains, such as polenta, couscous and pearl barley
- honey
- noodles, such as rice or egg noodles
- oils, such as cooking oil spray, extra virgin olive oil, sesame oil and vegetable oil
- peppercorns
- reduced-fat coconut-flavoured evaporated milk or reduced-fat coconut milk
- rice, preferably basmati and brown rice
- rolled oats
- salt-reduced beef, chicken and/ or vegetable stock (or make your own)
- salt-reduced tomato passata
- salt-reduced tomato paste (puree)
- seeds, such as poppy, sesame and sunflower seeds
- semi- or sun-dried tomatoes
- spices, such as chilli powder, cinnamon, cloves, cumin seeds, curry powder, dried chilli flakes, dried oregano, fennel seeds, ground allspice, ground coriander, ground cumin, ground turmeric, Moroccan spice mix, mustard seeds, nutmeg, smoked paprika, star anise and sweet paprika
- sugar or powdered sweetener
- tinned or dried beans, chickpeas, lentils and other legumes
- tinned tuna and salmon
- tinned unsweetened fruit
- tinned vegetables, such as artichokes, baby beetroot, bamboo shoots, corn kernels and tomatoes
- vanilla extract or essence
- vinegars, such as balsamic, cider, white, rice, white wine and red wine vinegar

## CONDIMENTS

- chilli paste
- fish sauce
- hoisin sauce
- green and red curry paste
- horseradish cream
- lemon juice
- lime juice
- mirin
- mustard: English, Dijon and/ or seeded
- oyster sauce
- reduced-fat mayonnaise
- salt-reduced soy sauce
- tomato sauce
- Vegemite
- Worcestershire sauce

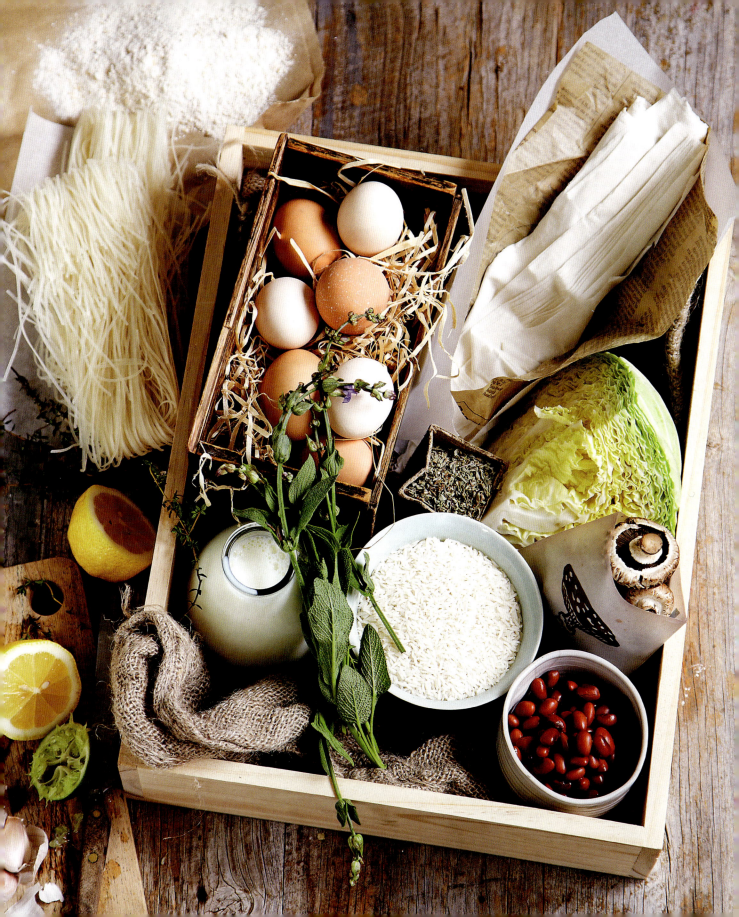

# growing your own herbs

Cooking with fresh herbs is one of the easiest ways to add flavour and interest to meals, but they can be expensive to buy, especially if you only use a handful and end up throwing the rest away. A great way to save money without compromising on flavour is to grow your own herbs. You don't need a backyard – herbs grow just as well in pots as they do in garden beds, so any sunny spot will suffice (a windowsill is perfect).

If you've never grown herbs before or are a bit of a reluctant gardener, just start with one pot (choose your favourite herb). Soon you'll have the confidence to add others to your collection. The following are all easy to grow and, if looked after, will provide a continual supply of fresh herbs to liven up your cooking.

## Parsley (flat-leaf or curly)

Parsley is an extremely versatile herb that goes well with almost any savoury dish. Stews, soups, fish, meatballs, salads, dressings, sauces and marinades are all given a fresh lift when a handful or two of chopped parsley is added.

It can be grown from seed or seedling, in a pot or in a garden bed. If you're new to growing herbs, parsley is a great herb to start with, as you can harvest the leaves as soon as the plant is established. Snip some leaves off every day to add to meals – in fact, the more you use, the denser the bush will grow.

Some recipes in this book that feature parsley:

- Lamb kebabs with spiced eggplant dip and tomato cucumber salad
- Steamed fish with fennel and orange salad
- Hearty vegetable soup
- Anchovy and parsley pasta sauce
- Salsa verde

## Mint

A pot of mint on the windowsill not only provides you with plenty of leaves to add to all manner of sweet and savoury dishes or to use to make a soothing cup of tea, it also emits a lovely sweet fragrance that will lift your spirits. Mint is available in many different varieties, and is a favourite in Asian and Middle Eastern cuisines. It tends to spread, so grow it in a pot to contain it, and water it regularly as it's a thirsty plant.

Some recipes in this book that feature mint:

- Roast cauliflower and lentil salad with chargrilled zucchini
- Garlic and mint pea puree
- Shaved cabbage, radish and fennel salad
- Roast beetroot, garlic and yoghurt dip

## Basil

The sweet peppery aroma of basil is a favourite in Italian cuisine, and its leaves can be stirred through all manner of pasta sauces to give an extra flavour burst. Crushed in a mortar and pestle, it is the basis for a versatile Italian pesto. Its pungent flavour is also wonderful in salads and is the perfect partner for tomatoes.

Some recipes in this book that feature basil:

- Slow-baked chicken with black olives, tomato and oregano
- Basil and olive pasta sauce
- Tuna burgers with blackened corn salsa

## Sage

Sage is a hardy herb that is a cinch to grow in a pot or in the ground. The soft, grey-green leaves are strongly flavoured and go particularly well with meat dishes and in stuffings.

Some recipes in this book that feature sage:

- Creamy chicken and mushroom soup with rocket pesto
- Garlic and sage chicken with squash and feta salad

## Oregano

Oregano is a Mediterranean herb that features heavily in Italian cooking. It will grow well in a large pot or in the soil, where it will spread as ground cover. It can be used fresh or dried in the kitchen; the dried leaves have a stronger taste.

Some recipes in this book that feature oregano:

- Oregano and lemon chicken with Greek salad
- Roast capsicum and tomato salad
- Baked ricotta with roast capsicum and tomato salad

## Thyme

A hardy plant that needs little water, thyme is a handy staple to have in your kitchen garden. Just a sprig of this aromatic herb thrown into winter dishes such as casseroles or soups, or sprinkled over roast potatoes, will add another dimension of flavour.

Some recipes in this book that feature thyme:

- Soft-boiled eggs with cheesy soldiers and baked mushrooms
- Braised beef, rosemary and mushroom casserole
- Braised lamb shoulder with roast fennel
- Chicken baked in a bread crust with lentil salad
- Fragrant chicken with pickled radish salad

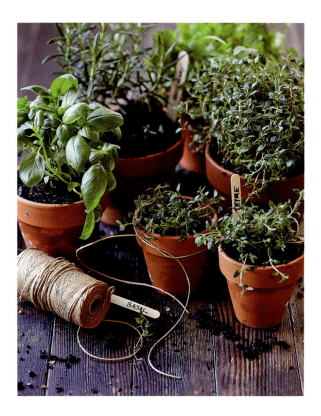

## Coriander

Coriander grows best in temperate climates, and can be planted in pots or garden beds. Its leaves look similar to flat-leaf parsley leaves, and they are often mistaken for each other, though coriander has a distinctive aroma and a much stronger taste. Pick the leaves as needed to add to stir-fries, soups and curries. The stems, roots and seeds can also be eaten.

Some recipes in this book that feature coriander:

- Coriander and vegetable soup
- Thai green curry paste
- Indian-spiced cauliflower and chickpea salad with blackened onions
- Moroccan-spiced lamb with lentils and roast pumpkin
- Thai-style san choi bao
- Shellfish curry with tomato and lemongrass

# BREAKFAST, BRUNCH & SNACKS

2 cups (450 g) chopped rockmelon
1 ripe banana
1¼ cups (310 ml) reduced-fat milk,
  reduced-fat soy milk or reduced-fat
  almond milk
125 g reduced-fat plain yoghurt
1 tablespoon honey
4 tablespoons bran flakes
pinch ground cinnamon
small handful ice cubes

# Breakfast smoothies

SERVES 2  PREP **5 mins**

**A complete breakfast in itself, a smoothie is a quick and easy way to get the day started with minimal fuss. This one combines rockmelon and banana – see below for two more delicious flavour combinations.**

1 Place all the ingredients into a blender and blend until smooth.

**Variations**

MANGO AND COCONUT: Replace the rockmelon with the flesh from one mango. Use ⅔ cup (160 ml) reduced-fat coconut-flavoured evaporated milk and ½ cup (125 ml) water in place of the milk.

MIXED BERRY: Replace the fruit with 2 cups (300 g) mixed fresh or frozen berries, and use reduced-fat strawberry yoghurt instead of plain. Omit the cinnamon.

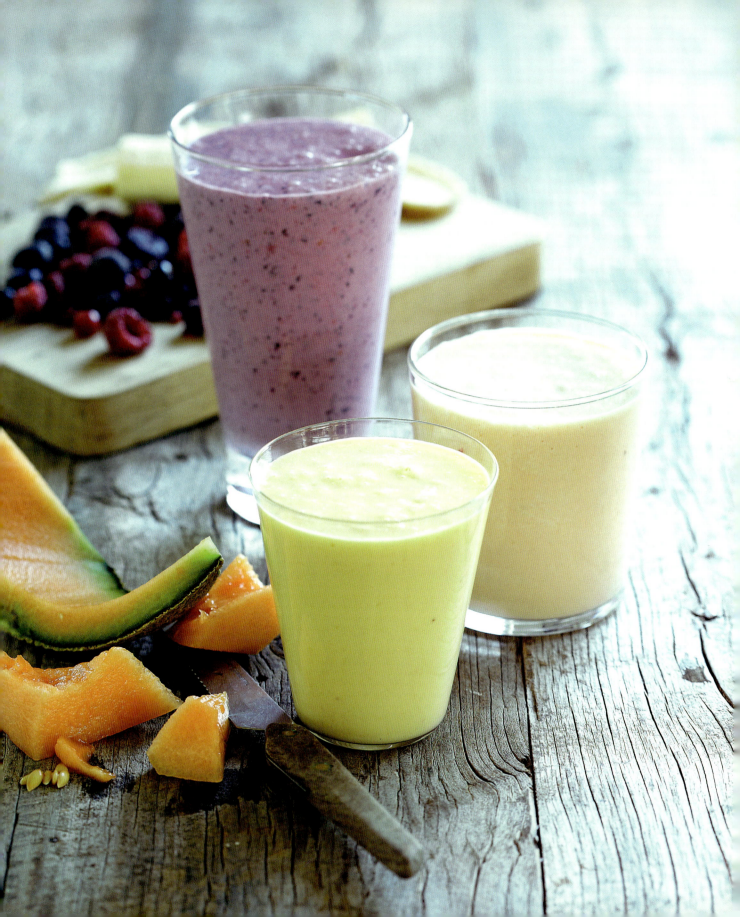

# Pear, strawberry and kiwifruit bircher muesli

SERVES 8 PREP **10 mins, plus soaking time**

1 cup (90 g) rolled oats
1 cup (110 g) untoasted muesli
1 cup (60 g) unprocessed wheat bran
2 tablespoons lemon juice
3 tablespoons slivered almonds or
   pistachios, toasted
1 green pear, coarsely grated
800 g reduced-fat strawberry yoghurt

**TO SERVE**
250 g strawberries, hulled and sliced
2 kiwifruits, peeled and chopped
2 tablespoons honey

**This bircher muesli is a delicious, healthy alternative to store-bought muesli. It needs to be soaked overnight before eating, or you could make up a whole batch at the start of the week and you'll have your breakfasts sorted.**

1 Place the oats, muesli and bran in a large bowl and pour over the lemon juice and 2 cups (500 ml) hot water. Cover and leave to soak for 30 minutes, then add the nuts, grated pear and 200 g of the yoghurt. Stir well to combine, then cover again and refrigerate overnight.

2 For each serving, spoon ½ cup (130 g) of the soaked muesli into a bowl, top with a couple of sliced strawberries and about ¼ of a chopped kiwifruit, then drizzle over a teaspoon of honey. Serve with 75 g strawberry yoghurt on top.

**Tip:** You can top your bircher muesli with any combination of seasonal fruit you like: try bananas, berries, mango or pineapple. Vary the flavour of the reduced-fat yoghurt for even more tasty options.

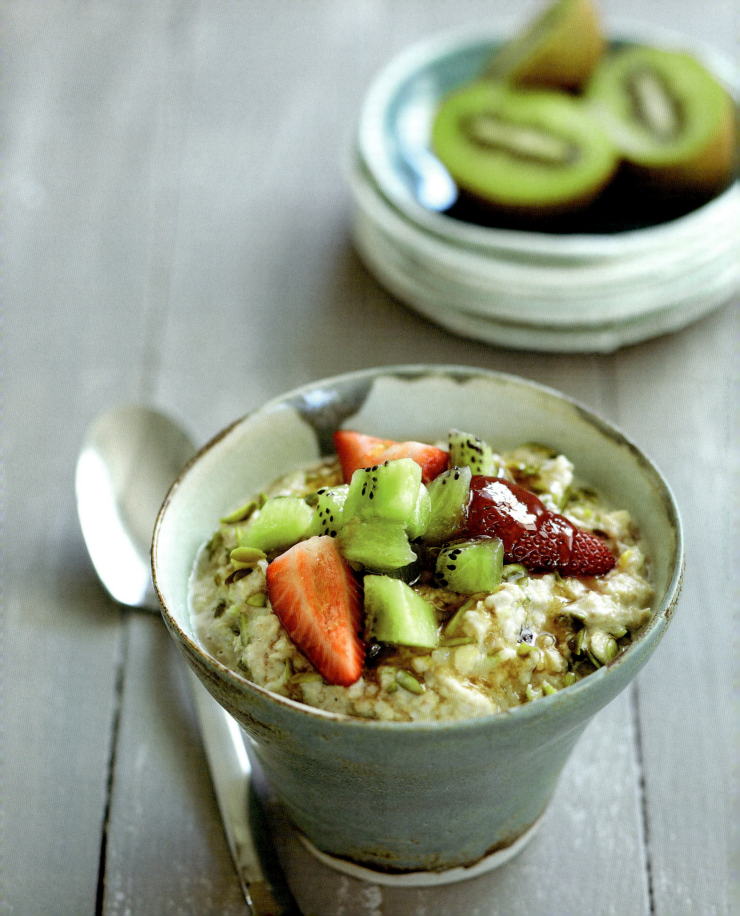

**1 SERVE (1 SLICE) =** ½ unit fruit
**2 units bread** ¾ unit fats

# Breakfast banana bread

MAKES 8 SLICES  PREP **15 mins**  COOK **1 hour**

**This bread is especially good lightly toasted.
Freeze leftover slices, individually wrapped
in plastic wrap, for up to 2 weeks.**

cooking oil spray
1¼ cups (200 g) wholemeal self-raising flour
¾ cup (110 g) self-raising flour
½ cup (12.5 g) powdered sweetener
1 teaspoon ground nutmeg
1 teaspoon baking powder
½ cup (125 ml) reduced-fat buttermilk
  or reduced-fat milk
1 egg, lightly beaten
1 teaspoon vanilla extract or essence
3 ripe bananas, mashed (you'll need
  1½ cups/360 g mashed banana)
4 tablespoons chopped walnuts or pecans

1 Preheat the oven to 180°C. Spray a 21 cm × 9 cm
  loaf tin with cooking oil and line with baking paper.

2 Combine the flours, sweetener, nutmeg and
  baking powder in a large bowl and mix well.
  In another bowl, whisk the buttermilk or milk,
  egg and vanilla together. Make a well in the dry
  ingredients and pour in the milk mixture. Stir
  in the mashed banana and chopped nuts.

3 Spoon the batter into the prepared tin and
  smooth the top. Bake for 55–60 minutes until
  lightly golden and a skewer inserted in the centre
  comes out clean. If the top is browning too much,
  cover with foil for the last 5 minutes of cooking.

4 Leave to cool in the tin for 10 minutes before
  turning out onto a wire rack to cool. Allow to
  cool to room temperature before slicing.

5 Store in an airtight container for up to 3 days.

**1 SERVE =** ½ unit dairy
**1 unit bread** ½ unit fruit

# Spiced ricotta fruit toast ›

SERVES 4  PREP **5 mins**  COOK **2 mins**

**The combination of ricotta cheese, cinnamon
and honey needs only toasted fruit bread to
make it sing. Use a sourdough fruit bread if
you have it.**

120 g fresh reduced-fat ricotta
½ teaspoon ground cinnamon
1½ tablespoons honey
4 slices sourdough fruit bread
1 mango, peeled and stone removed, flesh cut into
  cubes or 2 bananas, peeled and sliced
4 tablespoons fresh or frozen blueberries
½ teaspoon ground nutmeg, optional

1 Place the ricotta, cinnamon and 2 teaspoons
  of the honey in a bowl and mix until smooth.

2 Toast the bread and spread with the ricotta
  mixture. Arrange the fruit and blueberries on
  top and sprinkle with nutmeg, if using. Drizzle
  over remaining honey just before serving.

**Tip:** Use any in-season fruit you like: try strawberries,
peaches, nectarines or apricots.

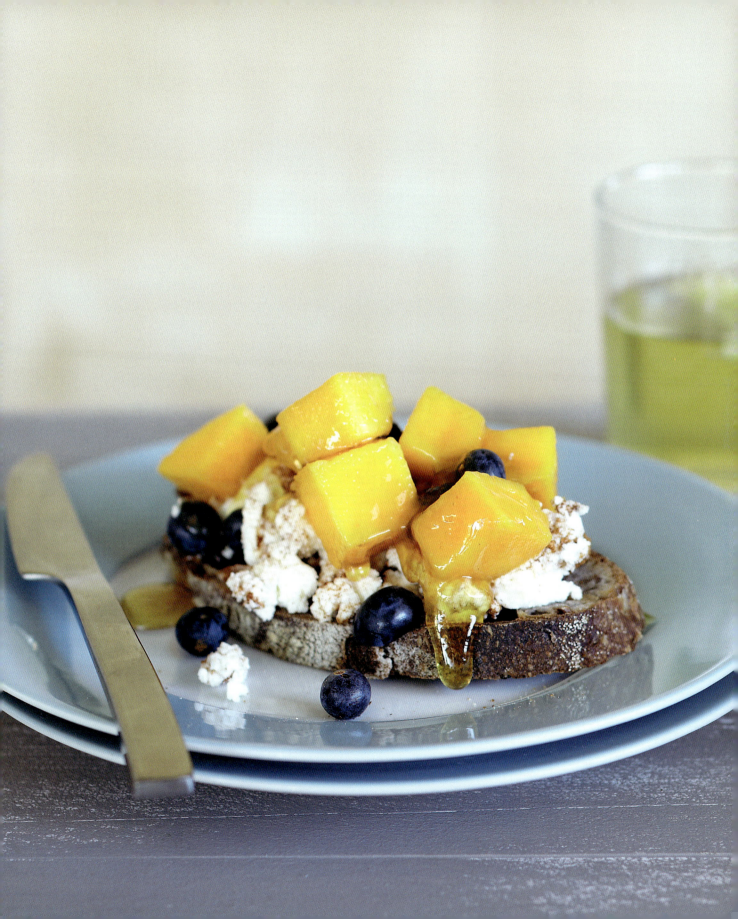

¾ cup (110 g) plain flour
1¼ cups (310 ml) reduced-fat milk
2 eggs
cooking oil spray

**CINNAMON-SPICED APPLES**
4 large granny smith apples, peeled,
    cored and sliced
3 teaspoons powdered sweetener
½ teaspoon ground cinnamon

**LEMON CURD**
²⁄₃ cup (160 ml) lemon juice
3 tablespoons caster sugar
1 egg, beaten
2 teaspoons finely grated lemon zest

**Tip:** To save time, you can prepare the
crepes the night before you need them.
Once they have cooled, wrap them
in plastic wrap and store them in the
fridge. When you're ready to eat, just
gently reheat them in the microwave
before assembling and serving.

# Lemon curd crepes with cinnamon-spiced apples

SERVES 4  PREP **15 mins, plus standing time**  COOK **40 mins, plus cooling time**

**A sweet treat for breakfast that will delight everyone. The cinnamon-spiced apples are really versatile and can be enjoyed in many different ways. You can prepare them in advance and store them in the fridge for up to 3 days.**

1 Sift the flour into a bowl with a pinch of salt. Whisk the milk and eggs together until combined, then whisk in flour until smooth. Cover and leave to stand at room temperature for 20 minutes.

2 Preheat the oven to its lowest temperature. Place an 18 cm non-stick frying pan over medium heat and spray lightly with cooking oil. Spoon 2 tablespoons of batter into the pan and swirl quickly to cover the base. Cook for 1–2 minutes until the underside is lightly golden, then flip the crepe over and cook for a further minute before transferring it to a plate in the oven to keep warm. Repeat with the remaining batter to make eight crepes.

3 For the cinnamon-spiced apples, place a saucepan over medium heat and add the apples, sweetener, cinnamon and ¼ cup (60 ml) water. Cover, reduce the heat to low and cook for 8–10 minutes until the apples are tender and the water has evaporated. Remove from the heat and set aside, covered, until ready to use.

4 For the lemon curd, place the lemon juice and sugar in a small saucepan over medium heat and cook, stirring, for about 2 minutes until the sugar dissolves. Remove the pan from the heat and allow the syrup to cool for 10 minutes. Pour the syrup into the beaten egg and whisk for 30 seconds, then strain through a fine-mesh sieve and return to the saucepan. Place over low heat, add the zest and cook, stirring, for 1–2 minutes until the curd thickens.

5 Divide the apple mixture among the crepes and fold over. Top each with 1 tablespoon hot lemon curd. Serve two crepes per person.

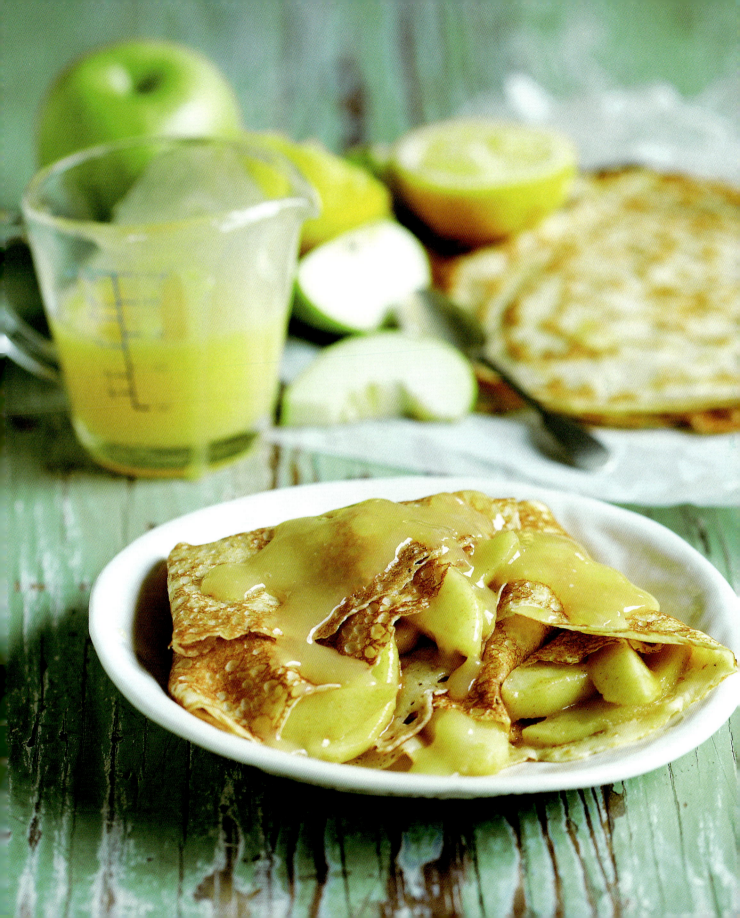

# Soft-boiled eggs with cheesy soldiers and baked mushrooms

SERVES 2  PREP **10 mins**  COOK **15 mins**

4 small–medium (about 150 g)
    field mushrooms, stems removed
    and finely chopped, mushrooms
    left whole
1½ teaspoons light margarine
½ teaspoon thyme leaves or
    finely grated lemon zest
1 tablespoon balsamic vinegar
4 eggs, at room temperature
2 slices wholemeal bread
50 g tasty cheese, grated
Tabasco sauce, to serve

**A perfectly cooked egg with a runny yolk is a beautiful thing. Make sure your eggs are at room temperature before you start, and set a timer for best results.**

1 Preheat the oven to 180°C, and line a baking tray with baking paper.

2 In a small bowl, combine the chopped mushroom stems with the margarine and thyme leaves or lemon zest. Place the mushrooms, cap-side down, on the baking tray and dot with the margarine mixture, then drizzle with balsamic vinegar and season to taste. Bake for 12–15 minutes until tender.

3 Meanwhile, shortly before the mushrooms are ready, bring a small saucepan of water to the boil. Add the eggs to the boiling water and cook for 4 minutes for a runny yolk (cook for a minute longer if you prefer a set yolk). Remove and place in egg cups.

4 Lightly toast the bread, then sprinkle over the cheese and drizzle with a few drops of Tabasco. Place under a hot grill until melted and golden, then carefully cut each slice into 2 cm thick soldiers.

5 Serve the eggs with soldiers and mushrooms alongside, and extra Tabasco if desired.

**1 SERVE =**
1 unit protein
1 unit bread
4½ units vegetables
½ unit fats

3 × 400 g tins chopped tomatoes
2 small red capsicums (peppers),
    trimmed, seeded and chopped
6 cloves garlic, thinly sliced
1½ tablespoons salt-reduced
    tomato paste (puree)
1½ teaspoons sweet paprika
cooking oil spray
8 large eggs
2 teaspoons Dukkah (see page 208)
    or toasted sesame seeds, to serve
2/3 cup (170 g) Zucchini Hummus
    (see page 204), to serve
4 slices wholemeal sourdough
    bread, toasted

# Israeli eggs with zucchini hummus

SERVES 4 PREP **10 mins** COOK **35 mins**

**Commonly known as shakshuka, this dish was typically cooked in small, individual frying pans to be eaten directly from the pan at the table. It's perfect to serve for brunch when friends drop over.**

1 Place the tomatoes, capsicum, garlic, tomato paste and paprika in a large saucepan, season to taste with salt and pepper and stir well to combine. Bring to the boil, then reduce the heat to low and simmer, uncovered, for 20–25 minutes until thick.

2 Spray two medium-sized frying pans with cooking oil. Ladle half of the tomato sauce into each one and bring to simmering point. Make four indents in the sauce and crack an egg into each one, then repeat with the other frying pan. Cover each pan and cook for 6–7 minutes until the whites are set but the yolks are still runny. Remove from heat and take directly to the table.

3 Spoon onto plates and sprinkle over the dukkah or sesame seeds. Serve with zucchini hummus and toast alongside.

4 eggs, separated
2 tablespoons chopped chives
50 g cheddar, finely grated
cooking oil spray
2 slices wholemeal sourdough
  bread, toasted

**SPICY GUACAMOLE**
½ avocado, seeded and sliced
1 tablespoon lemon or lime juice
4–5 drops Tabasco sauce
2 tablespoons finely chopped red
  (Spanish) onion

# Baked cheese and chive omelettes with spicy guacamole

SERVES 2  PREP **15 mins**  COOK **15 mins**

**Whipping the egg whites separately makes these oven-baked omelettes light, fluffy and a pleasure to eat.**

1 Preheat the oven to 200°C.

2 For the spicy guacamole, mash the avocado with the lemon or lime juice and a few drops of Tabasco until smooth. Add the chopped onion and season to taste, then set aside.

3 In a small bowl, mix the egg yolks and chives with a fork until combined, then season with pepper. In another bowl, whisk the egg whites with a pinch of salt until soft peaks form. Gently fold the egg yolk mixture and grated cheese into the whites, being careful not to overmix.

4 Heat a small ovenproof frying pan over medium heat and spray with cooking oil. When hot, pour half the mixture into the frying pan and tilt the pan to spread evenly. Cook for 2–3 minutes, shaking the pan occasionally, until the underside is golden. Run a spatula around edge of the omelette and fold over one half. Transfer the pan to the oven for 3–4 minutes until the omelette is cooked through. Gently slide it onto a chopping board and cover to keep warm, then repeat with the remaining mixture to make the second omelette. Serve with spicy guacamole and toast alongside.

**Tip:** If your frying pan isn't ovenproof, wrap the handle in foil to protect it.

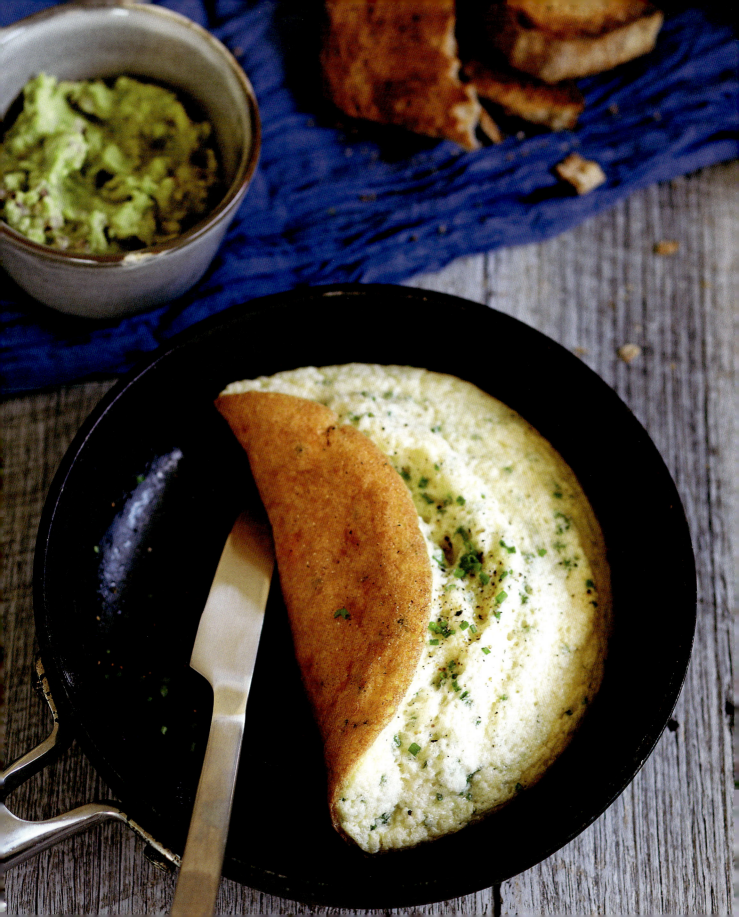

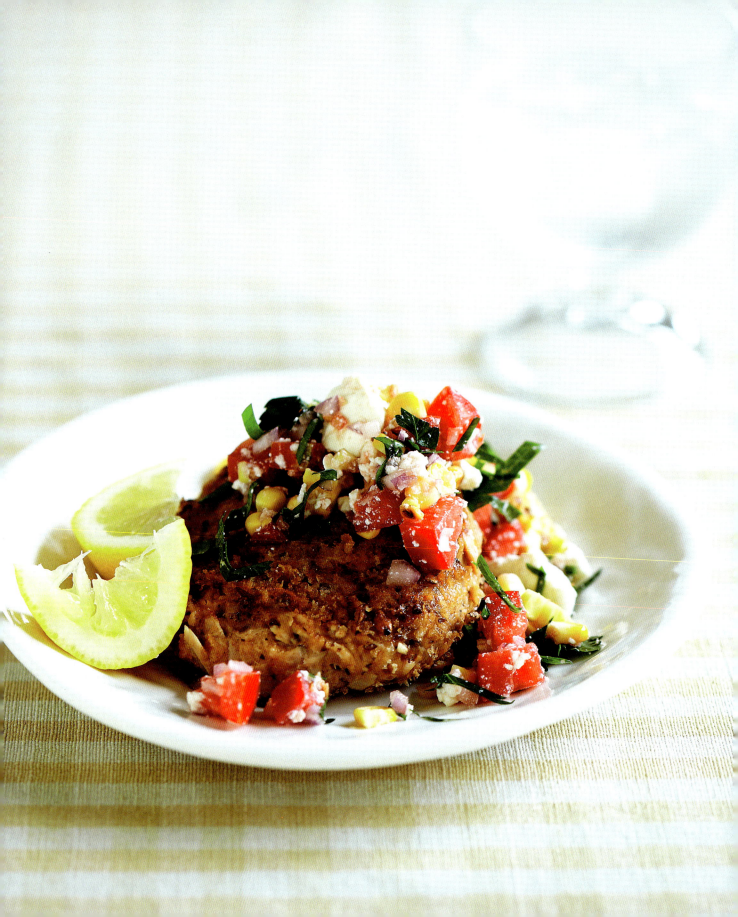

**1 SERVE =**
1 unit protein
¾ unit bread
¼ unit dairy
1½ units vegetables
1 unit fats

½ cup (35 g) fresh
  wholemeal breadcrumbs
300 g sweet potato, peeled
  and chopped
1 × 400 g tin tuna in spring water,
  drained and flaked
finely grated zest of 1 lemon
3 tablespoons
  reduced-fat mayonnaise
1 tablespoon Cajun Spice Mix
  (see page 208)
cooking oil spray
1 tablespoon chopped herbs,
  such as flat-leaf parsley,
  chives and basil
lemon wedges, to serve

**BLACKENED CORN SALSA**
2 corn cobs
cooking oil spray
½ red (Spanish) onion, finely chopped
2 tomatoes, chopped
1 tablespoon chopped herbs,
  such as flat-leaf parsley,
  chives and basil
60 g reduced-fat feta, crumbled
juice of 1 lemon

**Tip:** You can also serve these with
a green salad alongside to boost your
vegetable intake – see page 155.

# Tuna burgers with blackened corn salsa

SERVES 4  PREP **20 mins**  COOK **30 mins, plus refrigerating time**

**Prepare these burgers ahead of time, then cook them just before your guests arrive for brunch. You can prepare the salsa ingredients ahead too, just don't combine them until you're ready to serve. To make your own fresh breadcrumbs, remove the crusts from slices of wholemeal bread and process in a food processor until finely chopped. Freeze in plastic bags until required, and thaw before use.**

1 Preheat the oven to 180°C. Scatter the breadcrumbs on a baking tray and toast for 5–6 minutes until lightly golden.

2 Place the sweet potato in a saucepan of cold water and bring to the boil. Cook for 10–12 minutes until tender, then drain well. Transfer to a large bowl and mash. Add the flaked tuna, lemon zest, mayonnaise, cajun spice and half the breadcrumbs. Season to taste and mix well to combine. Shape into four patties, then place in the fridge for 20 minutes to firm up.

3 Meanwhile, for the salsa, heat a barbecue or chargrill pan to medium–high. Spray the corn with cooking oil and grill, turning often, for 8–10 minutes until cooked and blackened in spots. When cool enough to handle, place the cobs on their ends and carefully slice off the kernels, then transfer to a bowl and set aside.

4 Spread the remaining breadcrumbs on a tray and press both sides of the chilled burgers into the breadcrumbs to coat.

5 Place a frying pan over medium heat and spray with cooking oil. Cook the burgers for 3–4 minutes on each side until golden and heated through (handle them with care when turning them as they are quite delicate).

6 Add the remaining salsa ingredients to the corn kernels, pour over the lemon juice and season to taste. Mix gently to combine.

7 Serve the burgers topped with the corn salsa and lemon wedges.

cooking oil spray

200 g finely chopped lean,
   rindless bacon

2 zucchinis (courgettes), grated

2 cups (400 g) fresh
   reduced-fat ricotta

4 eggs

2 teaspoons thyme leaves
   or 1 teaspoon dried thyme

2 teaspoons oregano leaves
   or 1 teaspoon dried oregano

finely grated zest and juice of 1 lemon

¼ teaspoon dried chilli flakes

1 cup (70 g) fresh
   wholemeal breadcrumbs

80 g baby spinach leaves

Roast Capsicum and Tomato Salad
   (see page 154), to serve

# Baked ricotta with roast capsicum and tomato salad

SERVES 4  PREP **10 mins**  COOK **50 mins**

**Another great dish you can prepare ahead. Bake the ricotta the day before and store in the fridge in an airtight container, then simply bring it to room temperature before serving.**

1 Preheat the oven to 200°C. Spray a 20 cm round cake tin with cooking oil, then line the base with baking paper.

2 Heat a large non-stick frying pan over medium–high heat and spray with cooking oil. Add the bacon and cook, stirring regularly, for 6–7 minutes until crisp. Remove and drain on paper towel. Allow to cool.

3 Using your hands, squeeze out as much liquid as possible from the grated zucchini. In a large bowl or food processor, combine the ricotta, eggs, herbs, lemon zest, dried chilli flakes and half the breadcrumbs and mix until smooth. Stir through the zucchini and bacon and season to taste.

4 Spoon the mixture into the prepared tin and smooth the top. Scatter over the remaining breadcrumbs and spray the top lightly with cooking oil. Bake for 45–50 minutes until golden and a skewer inserted in the centre comes out clean. Remove from the oven and set aside to cool for 20 minutes before removing from the tin and slicing.

5 To serve, divide the spinach leaves among four plates and drizzle over the lemon juice. Top with some salad and two slices of the baked ricotta.

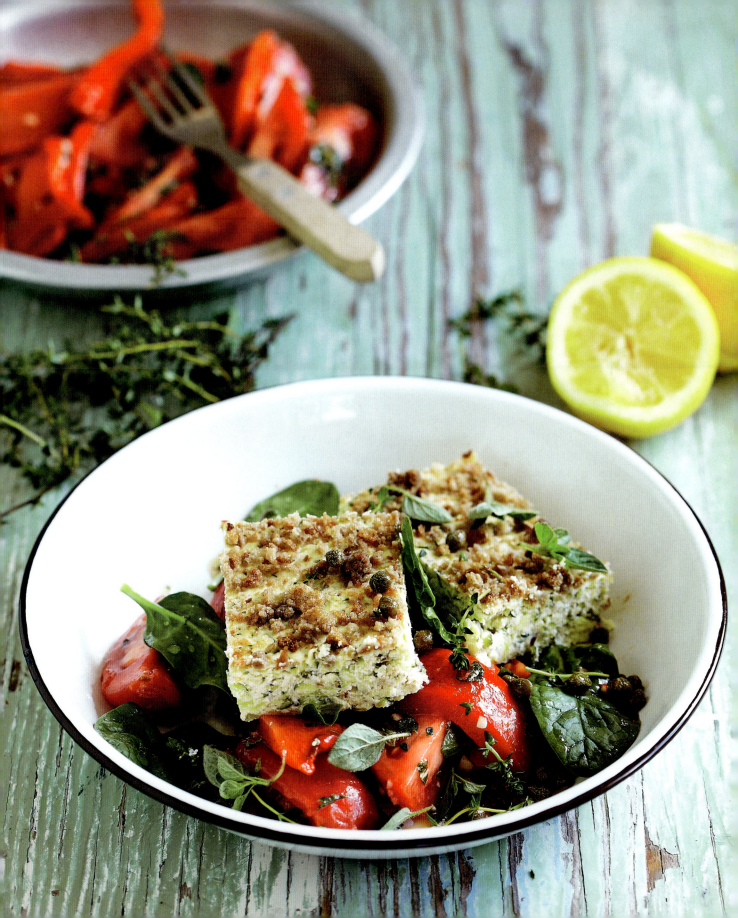

1 SERVE =
1 unit protein
1 unit bread
2½ units vegetables
1½ units fats

# Spicy baked eggs with cucumber salad

SERVES 2  PREP **10 mins**  COOK **30 mins**

2 teaspoons olive oil
1 onion, finely chopped
1 long red chilli, finely chopped
2 teaspoons salt-reduced tomato
  paste (puree)
1½ cups (375 ml) Slow-roasted
  Tomato Sauce (see page 198) or
  salt-reduced tomato passata
½ teaspoon cayenne pepper
cooking oil spray
4 eggs
4 tablespoons labna
1 tablespoon Dukkah (see page 208)
2 slices wholemeal bread, toasted

**CUCUMBER SALAD**
2 Lebanese (small)
  cucumbers, chopped
juice of ½ lemon
1 tablespoon chopped flat-leaf
  parsley or mint
2 teaspoons Dukkah (see page 208)

**A fiery way to start the day, these spicy baked eggs are rich and luxurious. Break the yolks at the table and stir through the tomato before eating. Labna is a creamy yoghurt cheese available from some supermarkets or specialty food stores – you can use plain yoghurt in its place.**

1 Preheat the oven to 180°C.

2 Heat the olive oil in a saucepan over medium heat. Add the oil and onion and cook for 7–8 minutes until the onion is soft. Add the chilli and cook for 2 minutes, then add the tomato paste and cook for 1 minute more. Stir in the tomato sauce or passata and the cayenne pepper, then season to taste. Bring to simmering point, then reduce the heat to low and cook for 5 minutes.

3 Spray 4 × 160 ml ramekins with cooking oil and place on a baking tray. Divide the tomato sauce among the ramekins. Make a well in the sauce and crack an egg into each one. Place the tray in the oven and bake for 15–17 minutes until the whites are set but the yolks are still runny.

4 For the cucumber salad, place all the ingredients in a bowl, season to taste and mix to combine.

5 Place two ramekins on each plate, spoon over the labna and sprinkle with dukkah. Serve with cucumber salad and toast alongside.

**Tip:** If you prefer a less spicy sauce, omit the cayenne pepper and remove the seeds from the chillies. You can use larger ovenproof dishes and cook two eggs per dish if you like.

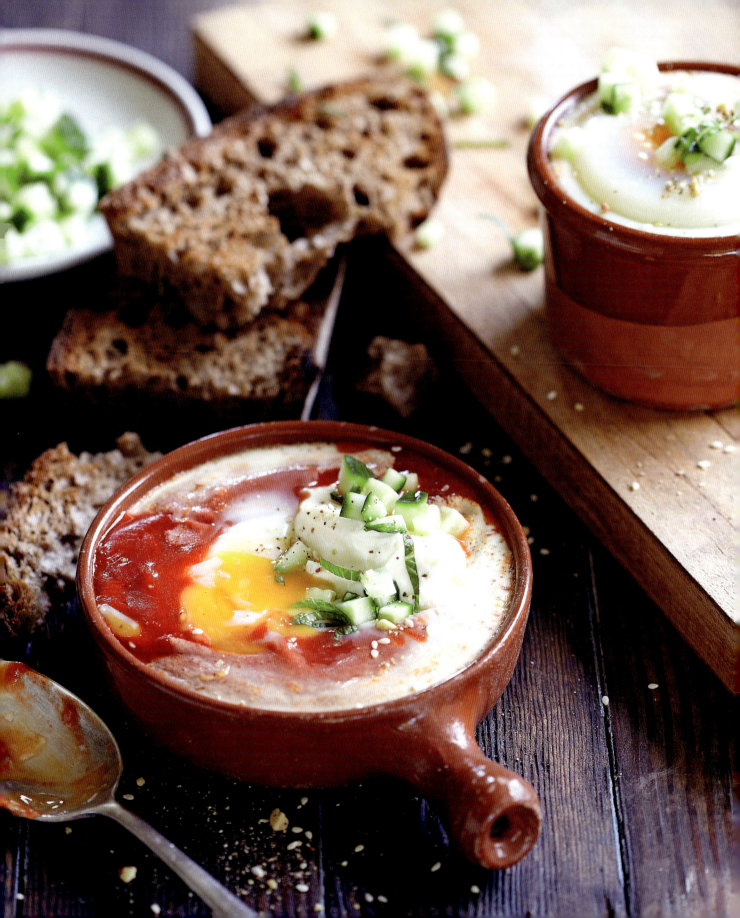

2 zucchinis (courgettes), grated
2 teaspoons olive oil
1 large red (Spanish) onion, halved, thinly sliced
1 teaspoon brown sugar
3 teaspoons balsamic vinegar
4 eggs
cooking oil spray
50 g feta
40 g baby rocket leaves
2 slices wholemeal bread, toasted

# Caramelised onion and zucchini omelette with feta

SERVES 2  PREP **10 mins**  COOK **25 mins, plus cooling time**

**You won't believe how sweet and comforting this simple omelette will taste. Caramelising the onions over low heat with the lid on will help to soften them and keep them moist while preventing them catching on the bottom of the pan.**

1 Using your hands, squeeze out as much liquid as possible from the grated zucchini.

2 Place a saucepan over low–medium heat. Add the olive oil and onion and stir well to coat. Cover with the lid and cook for 12 minutes, stirring every few minutes, until the onions are soft. Remove the lid, add the sugar and vinegar, then stir well and cook for 3 minutes.

3 Add the zucchini and cook for a further 1–2 minutes until the zucchini softens. Remove the pan from the heat and let the mixture cool for 5 minutes.

4 Preheat the oven grill to high. In a small bowl, whisk the eggs until combined. Add the onion mixture, season to taste and stir to combine.

5 Place a 22 cm frying pan over high heat and spray with cooking oil. Pour the egg mixture into the pan and give the pan a shake to distribute the ingredients evenly. Cook for 1 minute, lifting the edges of the omelette now and then to allow any uncooked egg to flow underneath.

6 Reduce the heat to medium and cook for a further 2–3 minutes until the underside is set but the omelette is still quite wet on top. Remove the pan from the heat, crumble over the feta and place the pan under the grill. Cook for 1–2 minutes until the omelette is puffed and golden. Run a spatula around the edges of the omelette and slide it out onto a chopping board.

7 Cut into quarters, then serve topped with rocket leaves and toast.

**Tip:** Keep a close eye on the omelette once under the grill as it will cook very fast.

½ **unit bread**
¼ **unit dairy**
¼ **unit vegetables**
½ **unit fats**

**cooking oil spray**
**1 tablespoon olive oil**
**50 g lean rindless bacon,**
  **finely chopped**
**½ red capsicum (pepper), trimmed,**
  **seeded and finely chopped**
**4 tablespoons wholemeal**
  **self-raising flour**
**4 tablespoons self-raising flour**
**2 teaspoons Cajun Spice Mix**
  **(see page 208)**
**4 tablespoons reduced-fat**
  **buttermilk or reduced-fat milk**
**65 g reduced-fat feta, crumbled**
**1 egg, beaten**
**1 × 125 g tin corn kernels, drained**
**2 tablespoons finely chopped chives**

# Cajun-spiced corn and bacon mini muffins (pictured overleaf)

MAKES 20  PREP **10 mins**  COOK **25 mins, plus cooling time**

**Sweet, slightly salty and studded with corn kernels, these mini muffins are a definite winner. Enjoy one as an indulgence or have two as a snack as part of your daily allowance (two mini muffins provide less than 450 kJ). Serve warm or at room temperature.**

1 Preheat the oven to 200°C. Spray 20 holes of a 24-hole mini-muffin pan with cooking oil.

2 Place a frying pan over medium heat, add the olive oil and bacon and cook for 4 minutes. Add the capsicum and cook for a further 2–3 minutes until it begins to soften. Transfer the mixture to a large bowl and leave to cool for 5 minutes.

3 Sift the flours into a medium-sized bowl, then add the spice and a pinch of salt and pepper and combine.

4 Stir the buttermilk or milk, feta, egg, corn and chives into the onion mixture. Make a well in the centre of the dry ingredients, then add the wet ingredients and mix until just combined. Spoon the batter into the muffin holes, filling each to two-thirds full.

5 Bake the muffins for 15–17 minutes until lightly browned, then leave to cool in the pan for 5 minutes before turning out onto a wire rack. Serve the muffins warm or at room temperature.

Tip: These muffins will keep for 2–3 days in an airtight container. Reheat by placing in a preheated 160°C oven for 10 minutes.

1 SERVE (2 MINI MUFFINS) =
¼ unit bread
¼ unit vegetables
¼ unit fats

cooking oil spray
1 tablespoon olive oil
½ small onion, finely chopped
4 tablespoons finely chopped red
    capsicum (pepper)
1 teaspoon dried Italian
    or mixed herbs
4 tablespoons wholemeal
    self-raising flour
4 tablespoons self-raising flour
½ teaspoon smoked paprika
4 tablespoons reduced-fat milk
50 g reduced-fat tasty cheese, grated
1 egg, beaten
2 tablespoons chopped black olives
1 tablespoon salt-reduced tomato
    paste (puree)

# Mediterranean mini muffins

MAKES 24  PREP **15 mins**  COOK **25 mins, plus cooling time**

**A couple of these muffins are an excellent option for a savoury snack as they provide less than 450 kJ, or enjoy one as an indulgence. Served warm, they taste just like a pizza, but without the calories.**

1 Preheat the oven to 200°C and spray a 24-hole mini-muffin pan with cooking oil (or line with paper cases).

2 Place a frying pan over medium heat and add the olive oil, onion, capsicum and dried herbs. Cook, stirring, for 7–8 minutes until the vegetables are soft. Transfer the mixture to a large bowl and leave to cool for 5 minutes.

3 Sift the flours into a medium-sized bowl, then add the paprika and a pinch of salt and pepper and combine.

4 Stir the milk, cheese, egg, olives and tomato paste into the onion mixture. Make a well in the centre of the dry ingredients, then add the wet ingredients and mix until just combined. Spoon the batter into the muffin holes, filling each to two-thirds full.

5 Bake the muffins for 15–17 minutes until lightly browned, then leave to cool in the pan for 5 minutes before turning out onto a wire rack. Serve the muffins warm or at room temperature.

**Tip:** These muffins will keep for 2–3 days in an airtight container. Reheat by placing in a preheated 160°C oven for 10 minutes.

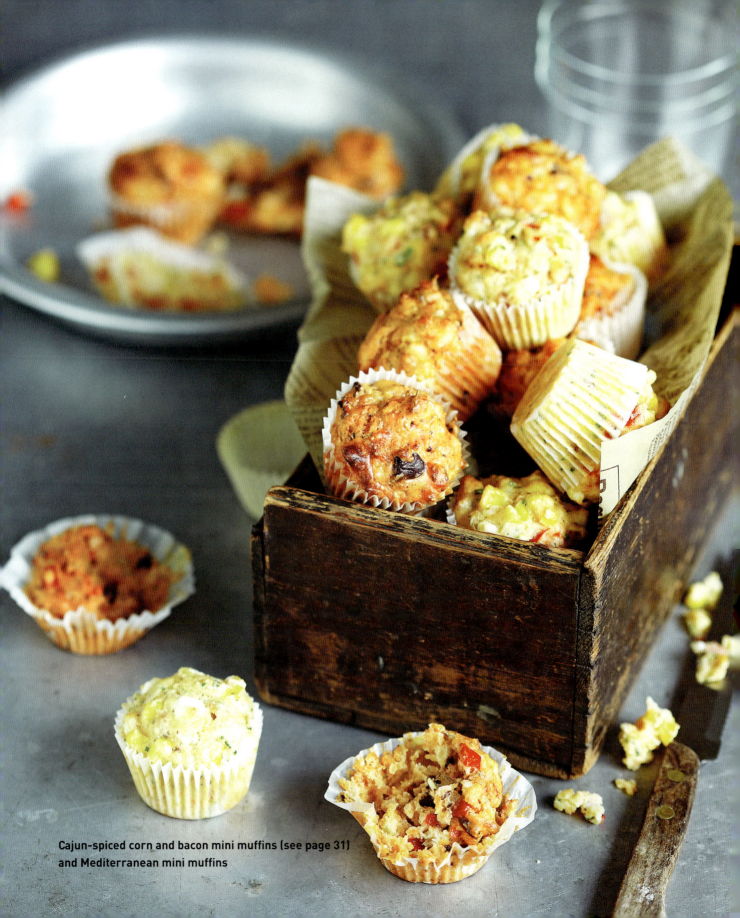

Cajun-spiced corn and bacon mini muffins (see page 31) and Mediterranean mini muffins

# LUNCH

**1 SERVE =**
1 unit protein
1 unit bread
2½ units vegetables
1½ units fats

# Asian-style tuna salad

SERVES 4  PREP **20 mins, plus soaking time**
COOK **8 mins**

**Light, fresh and loaded with herbs, this Asian-style salad is satisfying and won't leave you feeling heavy.**

4 tablespoons raw unsalted peanuts
2 cups (80 g) rice vermicelli noodles
2 carrots, cut into matchsticks or coarsely grated
2 zucchinis (courgettes), cut into matchsticks
1 red capsicum (pepper), seeded, finely sliced
4 spring onions, trimmed and finely sliced
1 × 250 g punnet cherry tomatoes, halved
1½ quantities Nam Jim Dressing (see page 206)
¼–½ head (150 g) iceberg lettuce, shredded
handful mixed herbs such as mint, coriander and basil
400 g tinned tuna in spring water, drained
1 long red chilli, seeded and finely sliced (optional)

1  Preheat the oven to 180°C. Spread the peanuts on a baking tray and roast for 6–8 minutes until lightly golden. Chop and set aside.

2  Meanwhile, soak the noodles in boiling water for 10 minutes until soft, then drain.

3  Place the carrot, zucchini, capsicum, spring onion and tomato in a bowl and toss with enough dressing to coat. Season with salt and pepper.

4  Toss the cooked noodles with 1 tablespoon of the dressing. Divide the noodles among four bowls, then top with the lettuce.

5  Arrange the vegetables on top of the lettuce, then flake over the tuna and sprinkle with the peanuts. Serve the chilli to the side, if using, along with any remaining dressing.

**Tip:** Use any kind of protein you have on hand. Firm tofu would work really well with these flavours.

**1 SERVE =**
1 unit protein
2 units bread
1½ units vegetables
½ unit fats

# Vietnamese chicken sandwiches ›

SERVES 4  PREP **10 mins**  COOK **10 mins, plus cooling time**

**Known as bahn mi, this classic French-influenced Vietnamese sandwich is traditionally served in a small baguette with pork. Replace the chicken with pork or prawns if you like.**

400 g skinless chicken thigh fillets, trimmed of fat
2 tablespoons reduced-fat mayonnaise
2 tablespoons hoisin sauce
2 spring onions, trimmed and finely sliced
4 iceberg or butter lettuce leaves
1 Lebanese (small) cucumber, thinly sliced lengthways
⅔ cup (60 g) Pickled Carrot (see page 201) or
    1 small carrot, grated
8 slices wholemeal or wholegrain bread
2 teaspoons salt-reduced soy sauce
finely sliced long red chilli and chopped coriander
    leaves, to serve (optional)

1  Bring a medium-sized saucepan of water to simmering point. Add the chicken and simmer gently for 10 minutes, then remove the pan from the heat and leave the chicken to cool in the water for 15 minutes. Remove the chicken with a slotted spoon and, when cool enough to handle, shred into pieces.

2  Combine the shredded chicken with the mayonnaise, hoisin sauce and spring onion and season with salt and pepper to taste.

3  To assemble, divide the lettuce, cucumber, chicken mixture and carrot among four slices of bread. Drizzle some soy sauce over each, sprinkle over the chilli and coriander (if using), then top with the remaining slices of bread.

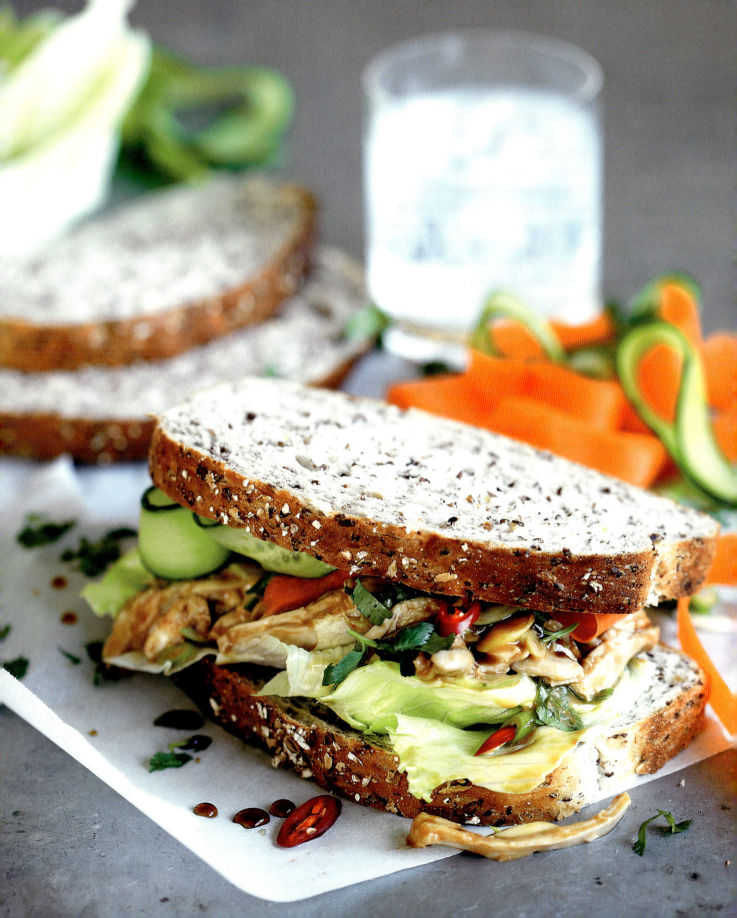

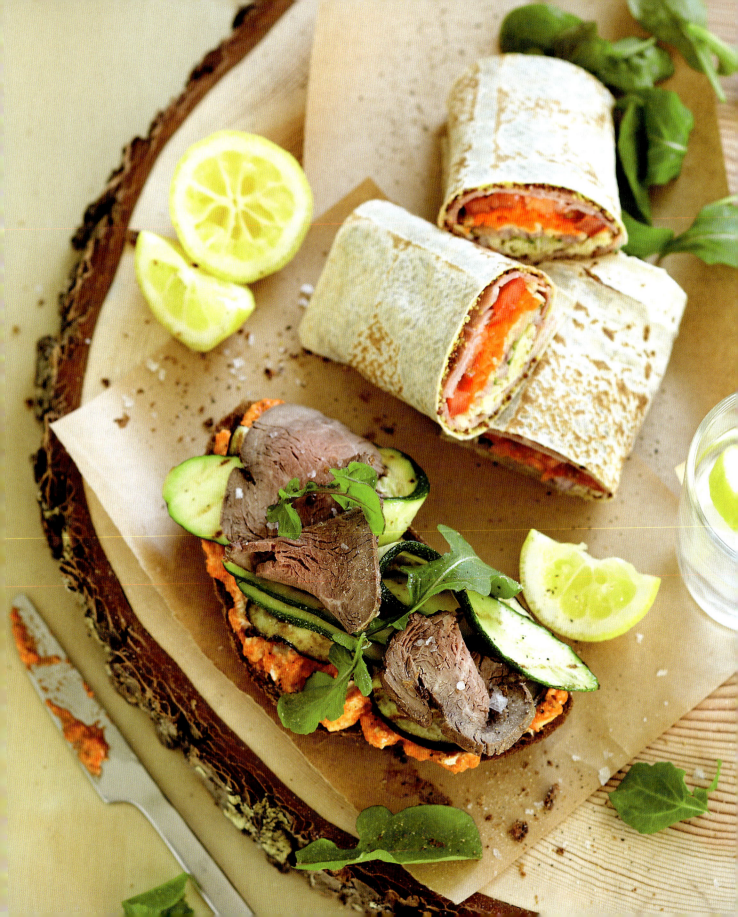

1 SERVE =  1 unit dairy
1 unit protein  1 unit vegetables
1 unit bread  ½ unit fats

# Roast beef on sourdough with chargrilled vegetables

SERVES 4  PREP **10 mins**  COOK **15 mins**

The addition of ricotta and romesco sauce elevates the humble roast beef sandwich to new heights.

1 small eggplant (aubergine),
  sliced into thin rounds
2 zucchinis (courgettes), sliced
  lengthways into thin strips
cooking oil spray
4 slices wholemeal sourdough bread
½ cup (120 g) reduced-fat ricotta
4 tablespoons Romesco Sauce (see page 196)
400 g leftover roast beef, thinly sliced
2 cups (80 g) watercress or rocket leaves
juice of ½ lemon

1 Heat a barbecue or chargrill pan to high. Spray the vegetables with cooking oil and, working in batches, cook for 2–3 minutes on each side until tender. Add the bread and cook for 1–2 minutes on each side until toasted.

2 Place the ricotta and romesco sauce in a bowl, season to taste and combine until smooth. Spread the mixture over the bread. Layer the eggplant, zucchini and beef on the bread, then top with the watercress or rocket. Squeeze over the lemon juice and serve.

**Tip:** If you don't have any romesco sauce on hand, substitute with 2 chopped roast capsicums. Fresh basil leaves and sliced tomato would also work well.

1 SERVE =  ¾ unit dairy
1 unit protein  1¼ units vegetables
1 unit bread

# Ham and cheese wraps with wholegrain mustard and pickles

SERVES 4  PREP **10 mins**

Pickled vegetables add pizazz to the classic ham and cheese wrap. This wrap tastes great toasted too – just cook in a sandwich press for 2 minutes until golden on both sides.

4 wholemeal mountain breads
4 tablespoons wholegrain mustard or English mustard
400 g lean, salt-reduced ham
1 carrot, coarsely grated
2 tomatoes, sliced
1 cup (150 g) Pickled Zucchini or Pickled Cucumber
  (see page 201)
¼ red (Spanish) onion, thinly sliced
120 g reduced-fat tasty cheese, grated

1 Spread each piece of mountain bread with 1 tablespoon mustard. Arrange the ham and vegetables on top, then sprinkle over the cheese and roll to enclose.

3 cups (750 ml) Chicken Stock
   (see page 209)
400 g skinless chicken thigh cutlets,
   trimmed of fat
1 tablespoon light margarine
2 leeks, trimmed, washed and
   chopped into ½ cm pieces
2 potatoes (300 g), chopped into
   small pieces
1 tablespoon dried sage leaves
300 g mixed mushrooms, sliced
325 ml reduced-fat milk

**ROCKET PESTO**
80 g baby rocket
2 teaspoons extra virgin olive oil
1 tablespoon lemon juice
1 clove garlic, crushed

# Creamy chicken and mushroom soup with rocket pesto

SERVES 4  PREP **15 mins**  COOK **30 mins, plus cooling time**

**Rich, creamy and livened up by the zingy rocket pesto, this soup tastes as good as it looks. Prepare a big batch as it won't last for long.**

1 Bring the chicken stock to simmering point in a medium–sized saucepan. Add the chicken and simmer gently for 8 minutes, then remove the pan from the heat and leave the chicken to cool in the stock for 15 minutes. Remove the chicken with a slotted spoon and, when cool enough to handle, shred the meat into pieces and discard the bones. Spoon out 2 tablespoons of the stock into a cup or bowl and set aside, reserving the rest of the stock in the pan.

2 Place a large heavy-based stockpot over a low–medium heat. Add the margarine, leek, potato and sage and cook, with the lid on but slightly askew, for 8–10 minutes, stirring regularly, until the vegetables are soft. Add the mushrooms and cook for a further 3–4 minutes. Add the stock from the saucepan, season with salt and pepper to taste and cook for 10 minutes until the potato is tender. Allow to cool for a few minutes, then blend with a hand-held blender until smooth. Return to a low–medium heat, add the milk and shredded chicken and bring to simmering point.

3 For the rocket pesto, blend all the ingredients together, along with the 2 tablespoons reserved stock, then season with salt and pepper to taste.

4 To serve, ladle the hot soup into bowls and garnish with pesto.

Tip: Add diced carrot or celery or some fresh thyme or parsley to the soup base for a different flavour.

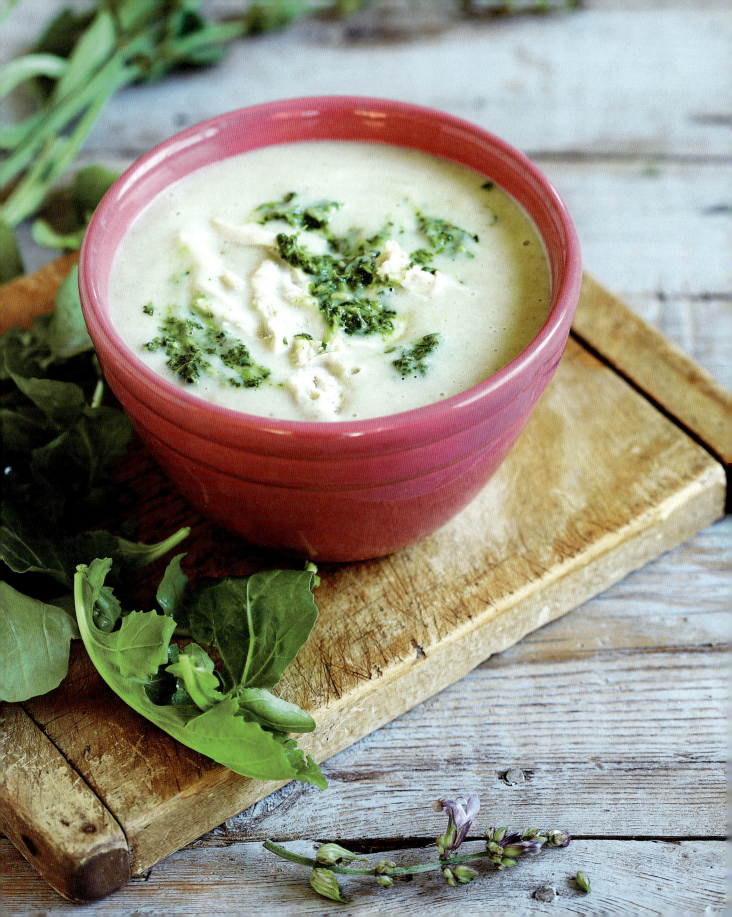

1 SERVE =   2 units vegetables
1 unit protein   1 unit fats
1 unit bread

# Tuna salad cups with paprika crisps

SERVES 4   PREP **10 mins**   COOK **7 mins**

**A quick and easy lunch to prepare ahead. Combine the salad and dressing but keep the paprika chips and lettuce cups separate until you're ready to eat.**

4 mountain breads
cooking oil spray
2½ teaspoons sweet paprika
1 × 420 g tin corn kernels
2 spring onions, trimmed and finely sliced
2 tomatoes, chopped
1 carrot, coarsely grated
2 tablespoons chopped flat-leaf parsley or mint
1 long red chilli, seeded and finely sliced
4 tablespoons reduced-fat mayonnaise
2 tablespoons lime or lemon juice
8 iceberg lettuce leaves, soaked in cold water
    for 10 minutes
400 g tinned tuna in spring water, drained

1 Preheat the oven to 180°C.

2 Lay the mountain breads on one or two baking trays and spray with cooking oil. Sprinkle over 2 teaspoons of the paprika and season with salt and pepper. Bake for 6–7 minutes until crisp. When cool enough to handle, break half into triangles and the rest into smaller pieces.

3 Place the corn, spring onion, tomato, carrot, herbs and chilli in a large bowl. Season with salt and pepper to taste, then combine well. Mix the mayonnaise, lime or lemon juice and remaining paprika together, then toss through the salad, along with the small paprika crisps.

4 Divide the salad among the lettuce cups, flake over the tuna and serve with the crisp triangles.

1 SERVE =   1 unit vegetables
1 unit protein   2¾ units fats
1½ units bread

# Mexican burrito wraps with guacamole ›

SERVES 4   PREP **10 mins**

**Wholemeal tortilla wraps are more flavoursome and earthy then the standard white variety. Make the guacamole as spicy as you like; just balance it out with an extra squeeze of lime.**

8 hard-boiled eggs, peeled, chopped
1 × 125 g tin corn kernels, rinsed and drained
1 × 125 g tin red kidney beans, rinsed and drained
3 tablespoons reduced-fat mayonnaise
2 teaspoons ground cumin
½ teaspoon smoked paprika
4 wholemeal tortilla wraps
80 g rocket leaves or any salad leaves

GUACAMOLE
120 g avocado
juice of 1 lime
3–4 drops Tabasco sauce (optional)
1 small tomato, chopped
½ red (Spanish) onion, finely chopped

1 Combine the eggs, corn, kidney beans, mayonnaise and spices in a bowl. Season to taste with salt and pepper, mix well and set aside.

2 For the guacamole, mash the avocado with the lime juice and Tabasco until smooth, then stir through the tomato and onion.

3 Spread each tortilla with ¼ of the guacamole, then top with the egg mixture and some rocket. Roll to enclose.

**Tip:** Replace the eight eggs with 400 g cooked chicken, pork or tinned tuna, if liked.

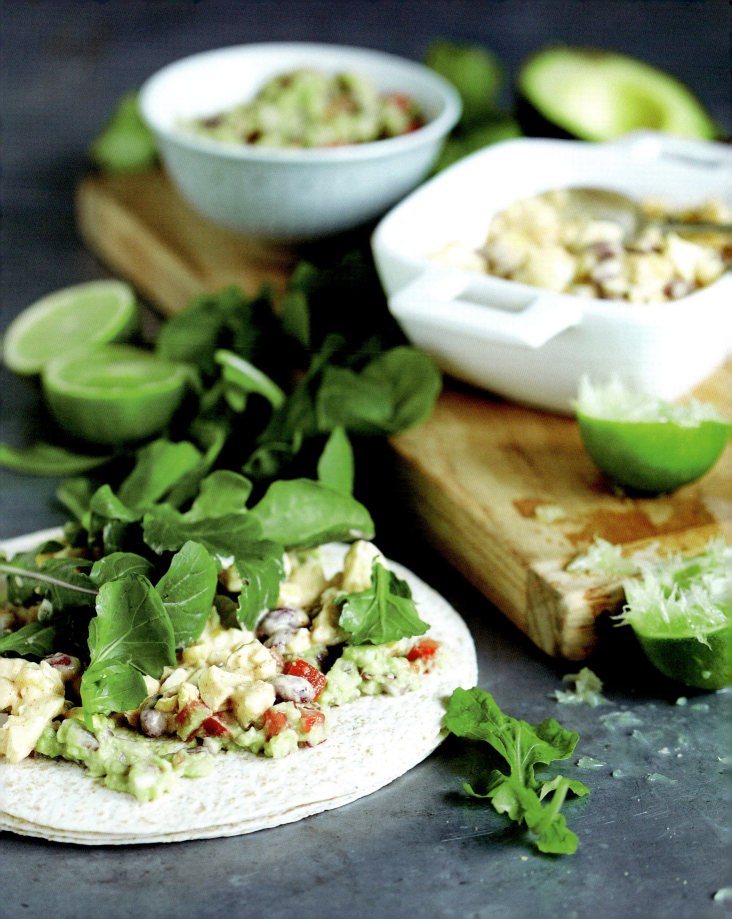

1 SERVE =
1 unit protein
1 unit bread
2½ units vegetables
¼ unit fats

# Roast cauliflower and lentil salad with chargrilled zucchini

SERVES 4  PREP **25 mins**  COOK **30 mins**

1¹/₃ cups (200 g) frozen broad beans

2 cups (400 g) French-style (puy)
  lentils, rinsed and drained

finely grated zest and juice of 1 lemon

300 g cauliflower, cut into florets

2 carrots, sliced into 5 mm
  thick rounds

1 red (Spanish) onion, sliced into
  2 cm thick wedges

cooking oil spray

1 teaspoon ground sumac

1 teaspoon sweet paprika

2 zucchinis (courgettes), cut on the
  diagonal into 1 cm thick slices

2 quantities Garlic Yoghurt Dressing
  (see page 207), to serve

handful mint leaves, roughly chopped

**The lentils in this recipe contribute a protein unit, making this beautiful salad a complete meal.**

1 Preheat the oven to 220°C and line two baking trays with baking paper.

2 Blanch the broad beans in a large saucepan of boiling water for 2 minutes or until tender. Remove the broad beans with a slotted spoon and transfer to a bowl of iced water to cool. Drain again, then peel and set aside. Add the lentils to the pan of water and bring back to the boil. Reduce the heat to low and simmer gently for 20–25 minutes until the lentils are tender. Drain, then pour over the lemon juice and zest and mix gently.

3 Meanwhile, combine the cauliflower, carrot and onion in a large bowl and spray with cooking oil. Sprinkle over the sumac and paprika and toss well to coat. Arrange the vegetables in a single layer on the prepared trays and spray with cooking oil again. Roast for 20–25 minutes, turning once, until golden and tender. Remove from the oven and set aside until ready to use.

4 Heat a chargrill pan to high. Spray the zucchini with oil then cook for 1–2 minutes on each side until tender.

5 Place the broad beans, lentils, roast vegetables and grilled zucchini in a large bowl. Add the dressing and half the mint, season with salt and pepper to taste and toss gently to combine.

6 Transfer the salad to a large plate or platter, scatter with the remaining mint and serve.

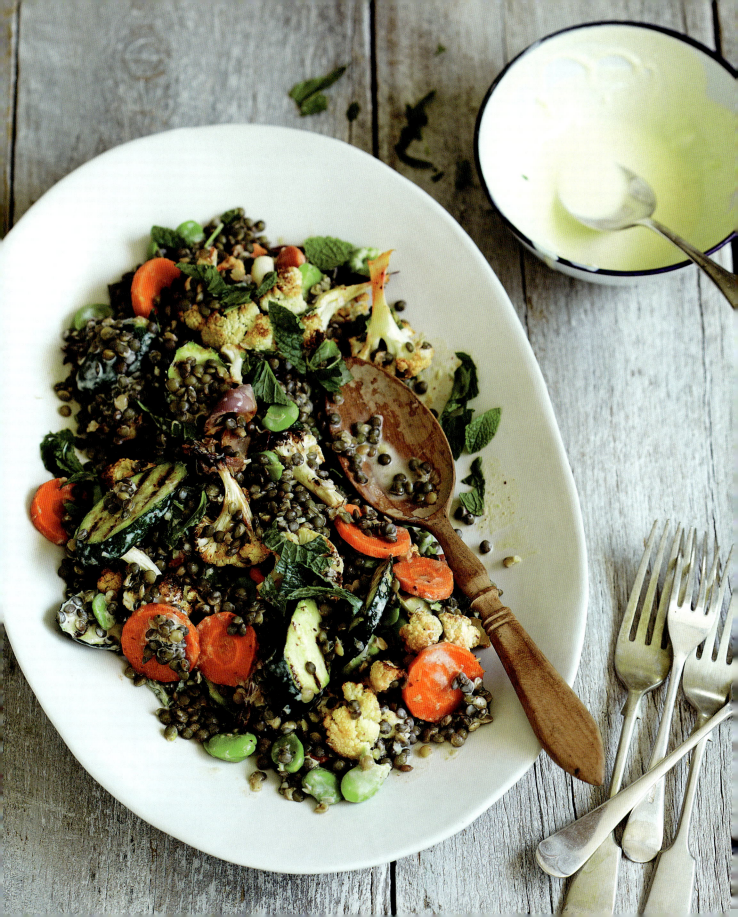

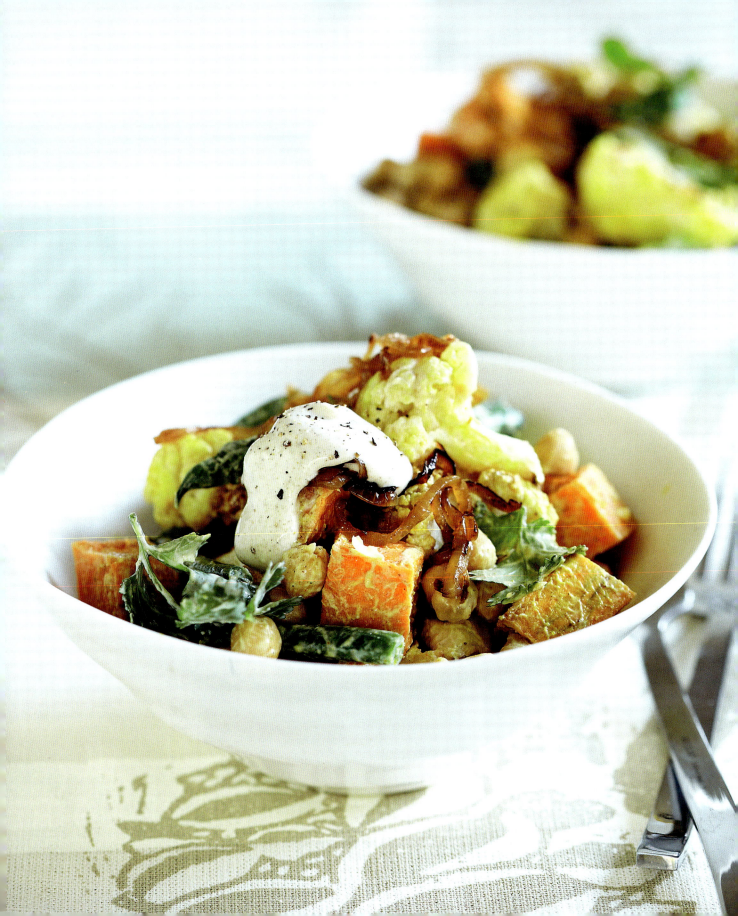

# Indian-spiced cauliflower and chickpea salad with blackened onions

SERVES 4  PREP **20 mins**  COOK **25 mins**

375 g cauliflower, cut into
    medium-sized florets
300 g sweet potato, peeled and
    cut into 2 cm pieces
cooking oil spray
1 tablespoon Garam Masala
    (see page 208)
1 teaspoon ground turmeric
1 tablespoon vegetable oil
2 onions, halved, thinly sliced
375 g green beans, trimmed
160 g reduced-fat Greek-style yoghurt
2 teaspoons ground cumin
juice of ½ a lemon
1 kg tinned chickpeas, drained
    and rinsed well
handful coriander leaves
lemon wedges, to serve (optional)

**Roast cauliflower is sweet and delicious. Teamed here with Indian spices and chickpeas, it makes for a hearty salad that is earthy and aromatic.**

1 Preheat oven to 220°C and line two baking trays with baking paper.

2 Combine the cauliflower and sweet potato in a large bowl and spray with cooking oil. Add the garam masala and turmeric and toss well to coat. Arrange the vegetables in a single layer on the prepared trays and spray with cooking oil again. Roast for 20–25 minutes, turning once, until golden and tender. Set aside.

3 Meanwhile, place a large frying pan over high heat. Add the vegetable oil and onion and cook, stirring regularly, for 8–10 minutes until the onions are blackened, then remove from the heat and set aside.

4 Steam or boil the green beans for 4–5 minutes until just tender. Drain, then refresh in cold water and drain again. Chop in half and set aside.

5 Place the yoghurt, cumin and lemon juice in a small bowl and combine. Season to taste with salt and pepper.

6 Place the roast vegetables, green beans and chickpeas in a large bowl. Add half the yoghurt mixture and most of the coriander, then toss to combine.

7 Divide the salad among bowls, top with the blackened onions and remaining yoghurt mixture and scatter over the remaining coriander. Serve lemon wedges to the side, if liked.

1 SERVE =
1 unit protein
½ unit bread
½ unit fruit
1½ units vegetables
1 unit fats

1 cup (150 g) frozen broad beans
1 tablespoon olive oil
1 leek, trimmed, washed and halved
   lengthways, then finely sliced
1 teaspoon fennel seeds
1½ carrots, coarsely grated
2 cloves garlic, crushed
4 × 100 white fish fillets (such as
   blue-eye, ling or snapper), skin
   and bones removed
finely grated zest of 1 orange
1 tablespoon chopped flat-leaf parsley
120 ml salt-reduced fish stock or
   white wine

FENNEL AND ORANGE SALAD
2 oranges, peeled and all white
   pith removed
2 tablespoons drained capers
1 bulb fennel, trimmed and
   finely sliced
1 tablespoon white balsamic vinegar
   or apple cider vinegar
small handful flat-leaf parsley leaves

# Steamed fish with fennel and orange salad

SERVES 4  PREP **20 mins**  COOK **25 mins**

**This is an impressive lunch to serve when you're entertaining. Use the fennel immediately after slicing, as it oxidises quickly.**

1 Preheat the oven to 180°C.

2 Blanch the broad beans in a large saucepan of boiling water for 2 minutes or until tender. Transfer to a bowl of iced water to cool, then drain, peel and set aside.

3 Cook the olive oil, leek and fennel seeds in a frying pan over medium heat for 3–4 minutes until the leek begins to soften. Add the carrot and garlic and cook for 3–4 minutes until soft, then remove from the heat and season with salt and pepper.

4 Cut eight lengths of foil about 40 cm long and place two pieces on top of each other. Fold in three sides, leaving one long side open. Repeat with remaining foil, then place the parcels on a large baking tray. Divide the leek and carrot mixture among the parcels and lay a piece of fish on top of each pile. Scatter over the broad beans, orange zest and parsley and season to taste. Pour a ¼ of the stock or wine into each parcel, then fold the open end over a few times to seal tightly. Cook in the oven for 12–14 minutes. Remove from the oven and check that the fish is cooked through: if not, reseal and cook for another 2–3 minutes before checking again.

5 Meanwhile, for the salad, segment the oranges by holding them over a bowl and using a small, sharp knife to cut the flesh away from the inner membrane, letting the segments and any juice fall into the bowl. Add the capers and fennel and toss to combine. Add the vinegar and parsley, season to taste with salt and pepper and toss to combine.

6 To serve, carefully open the parcels and transfer the contents to four plates. Spoon over some sauce and serve with the salad.

**Tip:** You can double the quantities of this recipe to serve for dinner.

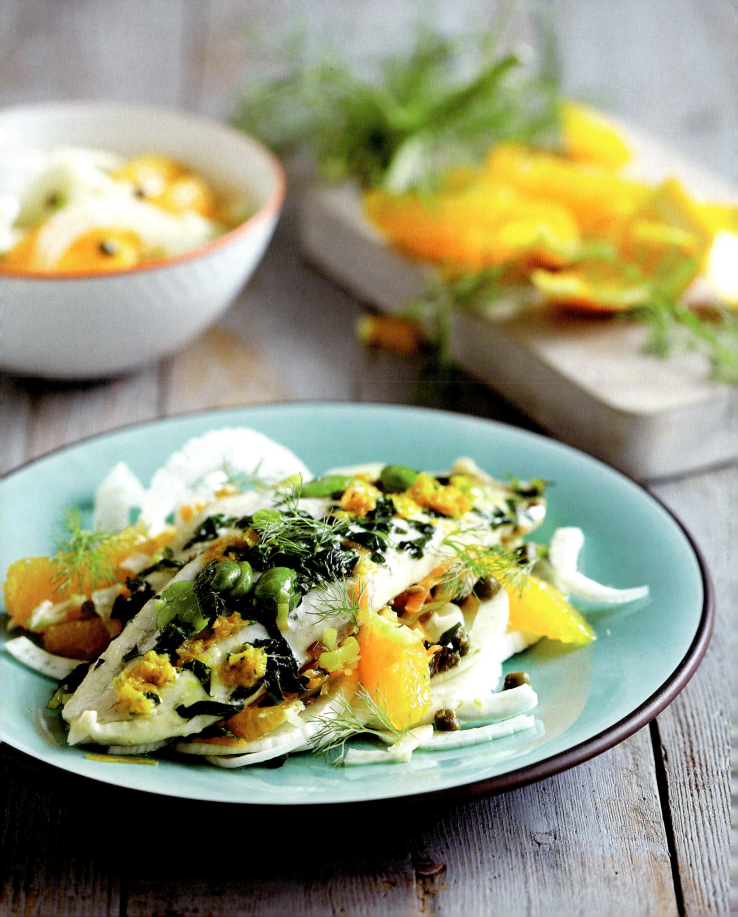

1 unit protein
¼ unit bread
2 units vegetables
1 unit fats

# Lamb kebabs with spiced eggplant dip and tomato cucumber salad

SERVES 4  PREP **20 mins**  COOK **8 mins**

400 g lean minced lamb
½ onion, finely chopped
3 teaspoons ground cumin
3 teaspoons ground sumac
1 teaspoon ground allspice
finely grated zest of ½ lemon
3 tablespoons fresh
    wholemeal breadcrumbs
handful flat-leaf parsley,
    finely chopped
cooking oil spray
Spiced Eggplant Dip (see page 202),
    to serve
lemon wedges, to serve

**TOMATO CUCUMBER SALAD**
3 tomatoes, cut into 1 cm dice
2 Lebanese (small) cucumbers,
    cut into 1 cm dice
small handful flat-leaf parsley,
    finely chopped
2 teaspoons extra virgin olive oil
juice of ½ lemon
½ teaspoon ground sumac

**Prepare the kebabs and eggplant dip the day before for a ready-made lunch. You can even cook the kebabs the day before too. Just wrap them in foil and heat gently in the oven when ready to serve. You'll need metal or wooden skewers for this recipe. If using wooden ones, make sure you soak them in water for 20 minutes before use.**

1 Place the lamb mince, onion, spices, lemon zest, breadcrumbs and ¾ of the parsley in a large bowl. Season to taste with salt and pepper, then mix with your hands to combine. Shape the mixture into eight even logs about 15 cm long, and thread these onto the skewers.

2 For the salad, place all the ingredients in a bowl, then season to taste with salt and pepper and toss to combine.

3 Heat a barbecue or chargrill pan to high and spray with cooking oil. Cook the kebabs, turning often, for 7–8 minutes or until cooked through.

4 Serve the kebabs with the eggplant dip and salad, with lemon wedges alongside.

Tip: Try serving the kebabs with Zucchini Hummus (see page 204) instead of the eggplant dip if you like.

1 SERVE =
1 unit protein
1¾ units vegetables
1½ units fats

500 g firm tofu, drained,
   cut into 2 cm cubes
cooking oil spray
1 tablespoon peanut oil
3 cloves garlic, sliced
2 tablespoons very finely
   chopped ginger
1 red (Spanish) onion, cut into
   1 cm wedges
2 carrots, sliced into thin batons
2 red capsicums (peppers),
   trimmed, seeded and cut into
   1 cm thick strips
2 bunches bok choy, cut into
   5 cm lengths, leaves and stems
   separated and washed
1 tablespoon Chinese chilli sauce
1 tablespoon tomato sauce
3 teaspoons salt-reduced soy sauce
2 teaspoons white vinegar
1 tablespoon toasted sesame seeds

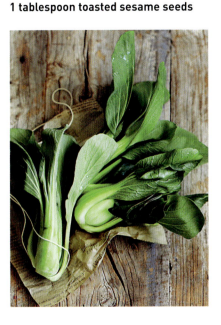

# Chilli, tofu and vegetable stir-fry

SERVES 4  PREP **20 mins**  COOK **20 mins**

**The secret to delicious tofu is to cook it until it is well-coloured on all sides – this will add flavour and texture to the finished dish. Chinese chilli sauce is available from Asian grocers, and be warned: it is very hot, not at all like its sweet chilli cousin. Use with caution, adding more to taste if you like it hot.**

1 Arrange the tofu cubes in a single layer on paper towel for 5 minutes to absorb any excess moisture.

2 Place a large non-stick frying pan or wok over medium–high heat and spray with cooking oil. Season the tofu generously with black pepper then fry in two batches for 4–5 minutes, turning carefully, until browned on all sides. Remove from the pan and set aside.

3 Increase the heat to high, add the peanut oil, garlic and ginger and cook for 1 minute. Add the onion, carrot and capsicum and stir-fry for 4–5 minutes until the vegetables begin to soften. Add the bok choy stems and cook for 2 minutes. Combine the sauces and vinegar, then add to the pan along with the bok choy leaves and the tofu. Toss gently for 1 minute until the tofu is heated through and the bok choy wilts.

4 Divide the vegetables and tofu among plates and sprinkle with the sesame seeds before serving.

Tip: Serve this with rice from your daily allowance if you like.

# Ginger-steamed tofu with stir-fried vegetables

SERVES 4  PREP **20 mins**  COOK **10 mins**

3 teaspoons peanut oil

1 tablespoon finely sliced ginger

1 long red chilli, sliced

2 red capsicums (peppers), trimmed,
   seeded and thinly sliced

150 g green beans, trimmed,
   halved lengthways

1 bunch bok choy, chopped into
   5 cm lengths, leaves and stems
   separated and washed

2 tablespoons oyster sauce

3 teaspoons salt-reduced soy sauce

**GINGER-STEAMED TOFU**

700 g silken tofu, drained, cut
   crossways into 3 cm thick pieces

1 teaspoon sesame oil

1 × 2 cm piece ginger, peeled and
   sliced into thin matchsticks

1 small red chilli, finely sliced

2 spring onions, trimmed and
   finely sliced

3 teaspoons salt-reduced soy sauce

**This dish features silken tofu, which has a soft, velvety texture, and is perfect for steaming.**

1 For the ginger-steamed tofu, arrange the tofu on a plate that fits inside a steamer basket. Drizzle with sesame oil and scatter over the ginger, chilli and ½ of the spring onion. Season with white pepper.

2 Half-fill a large saucepan with water and bring to the boil. Place the plate inside the steamer basket, cover and steam the tofu for 4 minutes, then remove from the heat and set aside.

3 Meanwhile, heat the peanut oil in a wok or a large frying pan over high heat. Add the ginger and chilli and stir-fry for 1 minute. Add the capsicum, green beans and bok choy stems and cook for 3 minutes, then add the oyster and soy sauce and cook for 2–3 minutes more until the vegetables are almost tender. Add the bok choy leaves and toss for a further minute until the leaves wilt.

4 Remove the plate from the steamer basket and gently drain away the liquid around the tofu. Spoon over the soy sauce and scatter with the remaining spring onion.

5 Serve the steamed tofu with the stir-fried vegetables.

Tip: Prepare everything before you start, as this will take no time at all to cook. Steam the tofu in a large wok with a stand if you don't have a steamer basket big enough.

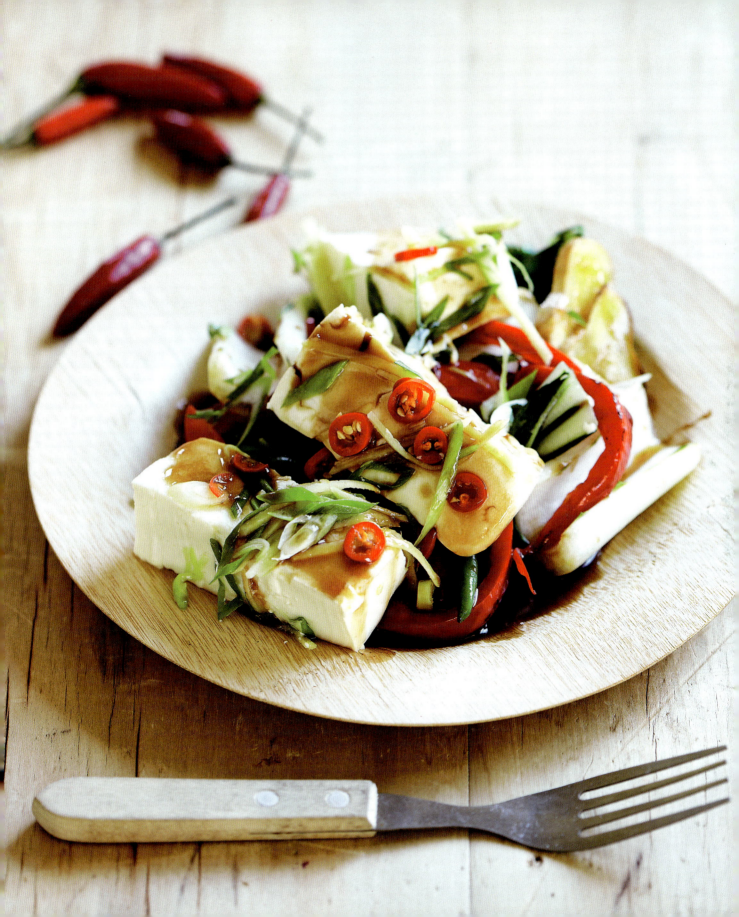

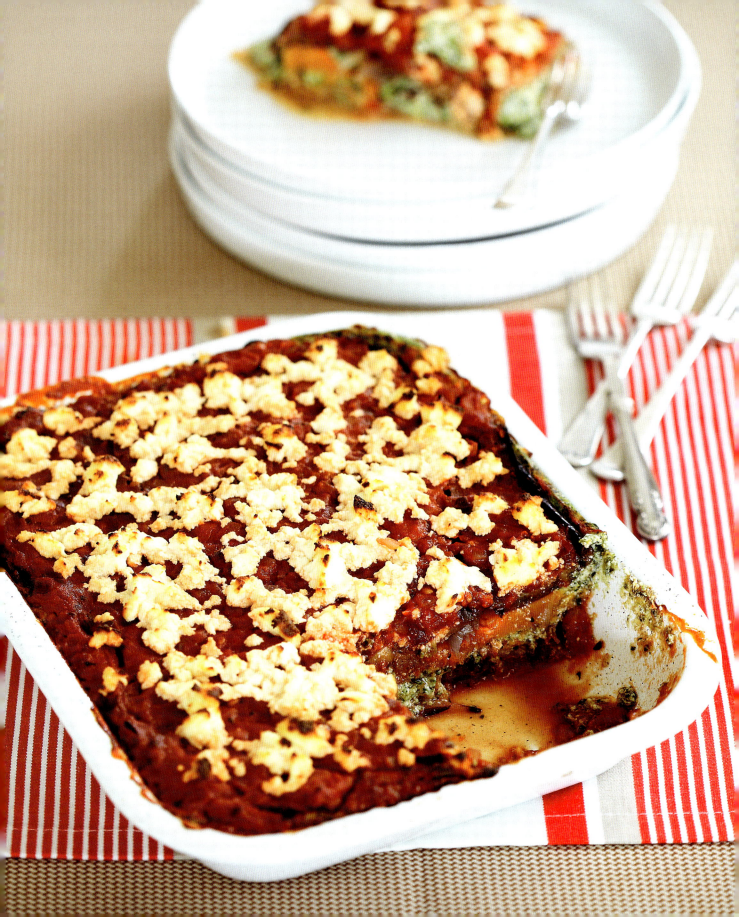

1 SERVE =
1 unit protein
½ unit dairy
3 units vegetables
¾ unit fat

# Roast vegetable and tofu lasagne

SERVES 6  PREP **25 mins**  COOK **1 hour**

1 eggplant (aubergine), cut
  lengthways into 5 mm thick slices
1 red capsicum (pepper), trimmed,
  seeded and cut into 1 cm thick slices
400 g pumpkin (squash), peeled and
  cut into 1 cm thick slices
2 red (Spanish) onions, 1 cut into
  1 cm wedges, 1 finely chopped
cooking oil spray
1 tablespoon olive oil
3 cloves garlic, finely chopped
2 tablespoons dried mixed herbs
2 × 400 g tins peeled tomatoes
2 tablespoons salt-reduced tomato
  paste (puree)
1050 g silken tofu, drained
180 g frozen spinach, thawed,
  finely chopped
100 g fresh reduced-fat ricotta

**A new take on an old favourite, this dish features roast vegetables, which add a lovely depth of flavour, and has creamy tofu masquerading as cheese (no one will know if you don't tell them!).**

1 Preheat the oven to 220°C and line two baking trays with baking paper.

2 Arrange the eggplant, capsicum, pumpkin and onion wedges on the prepared trays, spray with cooking oil, season to taste with salt and pepper and roast for 20–25 minutes, turning halfway through, until tender. Remove from the oven and set aside. Reduce the oven temperature to 200°C.

3 Meanwhile, place a medium-sized saucepan over medium–high heat. Add the olive oil, finely chopped onion, garlic and mixed herbs and cook for 4–5 minutes until the onion softens. Add the tomatoes and tomato paste and season to taste with salt and pepper. Bring to the boil, then reduce the heat and simmer for 10 minutes until thickened.

4 Blend the tofu and spinach in a food processor until smooth. Alternatively, place in a bowl and mix together by hand until smooth. Season to taste with salt and pepper. Roughly chop the roast onion wedges and stir through the tofu mixture.

5 Spray a 2.5 litre ovenproof dish with cooking oil. Pour half of the tomato sauce into the prepared dish. Arrange half the vegetables on top, then cover with the tofu mixture. Add the remaining vegetables, then top with a final layer of tomato sauce. Scatter over the ricotta and bake for 30–35 minutes until the ricotta is lightly golden.

**Tip:** Use any vegetables you have to hand in the tomato mixture, such as mushrooms, zucchini or celery.

1 unit protein
2 units bread
2 units vegetables
1 unit fats

# Gourmet vegetarian burgers

SERVES 4   PREP **25 mins, plus resting time**   COOK **30 mins**

1 cup (70 g) wholemeal breadcrumbs
1 bulb fennel, trimmed and cut into
    3 mm thick slices, fronds reserved
    and finely chopped
cooking oil spray
3½ teaspoons ground sumac
1 kg tinned chickpeas, drained
    and rinsed
finely grated zest and juice of 1 lemon
2 teaspoons dried mint
1 tablespoon extra virgin olive oil
¼ teaspoon chilli powder
2 cups (80 g) rocket leaves
    or watercress
2 tomatoes, sliced into
    1 cm thick rounds
8 tablespoons Zucchini Hummus
    (see page 204)
Honey-roasted Carrots with Cumin
    and Caraway (see page 146)

**Some of the best meat-free burgers you'll ever eat, these chickpea versions are not only seriously tasty, but they look amazing too.**

1  Preheat the oven to 200°C.

2  Toast the breadcrumbs on a baking tray for 3–5 minutes until lightly golden.

3  Arrange the fennel slices on a baking-paper-lined tray and spray with cooking oil. Sprinkle over ½ teaspoon of the sumac and season to taste with salt and pepper. Roast for 30–35 minutes until golden and crisp.

4  Meanwhile, blend the chickpeas in a food processor until smooth. Add the chopped fennel fronds, lemon zest, 2 tablespoons of the lemon juice, the remaining sumac, the mint, olive oil, chilli powder and 1 tablespoon water. Blend until well combined, then add the breadcrumbs, season to taste with salt and pepper and blend again. Taste, and add more lemon juice or chilli powder, if desired. Set aside for 15 minutes to allow the breadcrumbs to absorb some of the moisture. Divide the mixture into four equal portions and shape into 10 cm round burgers.

5  Place a large frying pan over medium heat and spray with cooking oil. Cook the burgers for 4 minutes on each side until golden and cooked through.

6  To serve, divide the fennel slices among plates, top with some rocket, a chickpea burger, tomato slices and zucchini hummus. Serve with cumin and caraway carrots alongside.

Tip: Prepare the burgers the day before and store covered in the fridge until ready to cook.

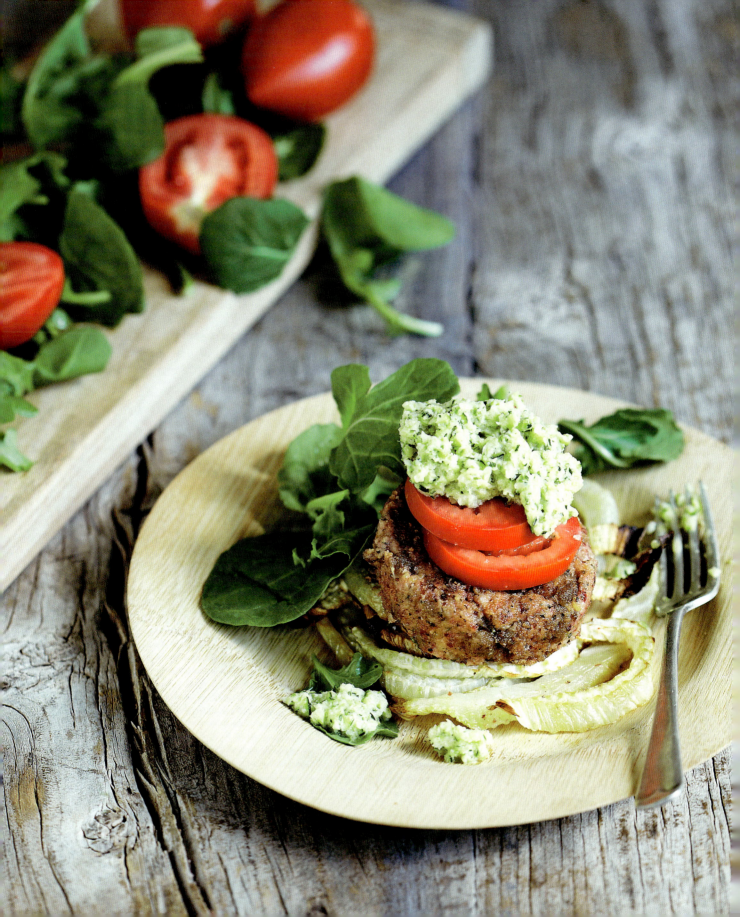

# BEEF, LAMB' & PORK

# Lemongrass and chilli barbecued pork with stir-fried vegetables

SERVES 4  PREP **15 mins, plus soaking and marinating time**
COOK **15 mins**

4 × 200 g barbecue pork chops
   (loin or blade), trimmed of fat
cooking oil spray
10 dried shiitake mushrooms,
   soaked in 1½ cups (375 ml) hot
   water for 20 minutes
3 teaspoons salt-reduced soy sauce
1 tablespoon fish sauce
1 tablespoon peanut or vegetable oil
1 stalk lemongrass, trimmed and
   finely chopped
2 cloves garlic, finely chopped
1 long red chilli, finely sliced
1 carrot, sliced into thin rounds
150 g snowpeas (mange-tout),
   trimmed
150 g green beans, trimmed and
   halved lengthways
4 spring onions, trimmed and sliced
   into 3 cm lengths
lime wedges, to serve (optional)

**LEMONGRASS AND CHILLI PASTE**
2 spring onions, trimmed and chopped
1 stalk lemongrass, trimmed
   and chopped
2 cloves garlic, chopped
1 long red chilli, chopped
1 tablespoon fish sauce

**Marinating the pork overnight not only adds flavour but also tenderises the meat. Even a few hours will make a big difference, so get started on the pork as early as you can.**

1 To make the paste, blend all the ingredients to a coarse paste and season with pepper. Rub the paste into the pork chops and marinate overnight.

2 Heat a barbecue or chargrill pan to high. Spray the chops with cooking oil and cook for 3–4 minutes each side until just cooked through. Cover with foil and set aside to rest for 5 minutes.

3 While the pork is resting, drain the mushrooms, reserving the soaking water, and slice thickly. Measure out 4 tablespoons of the soaking water into a jug, being careful not to get any of the sediment from the bottom, then mix this with the soy and fish sauces and set aside.

4 Place a large wok or frying pan over high heat. Add the oil, lemongrass, garlic and chilli and cook for 1 minute. Add the carrot and cook for 1 minute before adding the snowpeas, beans and spring onion. Toss and cook the vegetables for 1 minute, then pour in the sauce and toss quickly to combine. Cover and cook for 3–4 minutes until the vegetables are tender, then season with pepper.

5 Serve the pork chops and vegetable stir-fry with lime wedges alongside, if liked.

Tip: If time is short, serve the pork with steamed Asian greens dressed simply with fish sauce and lemon juice.

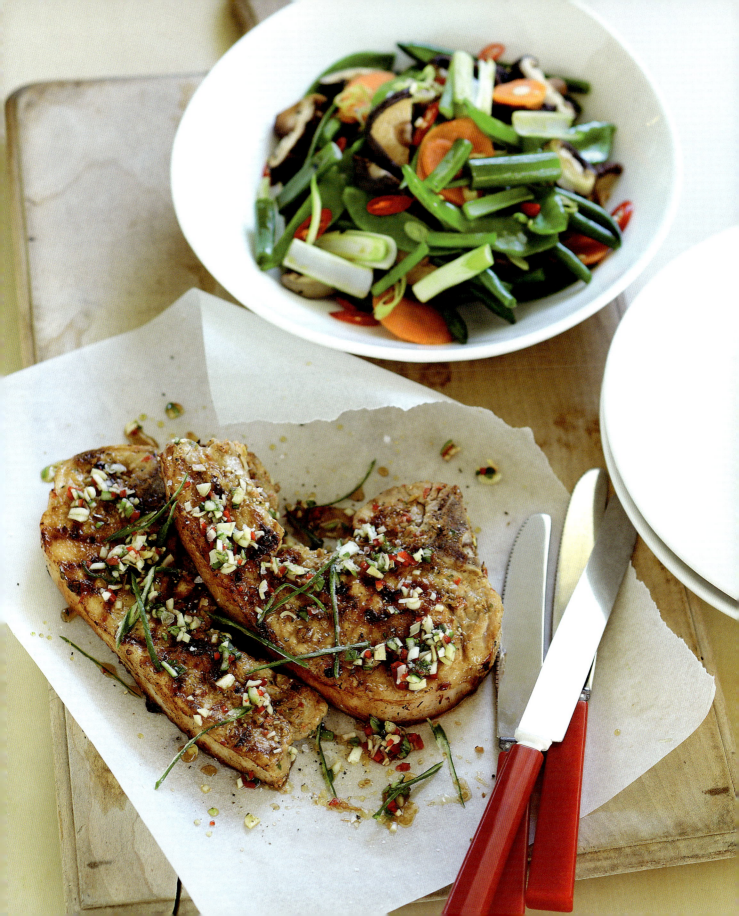

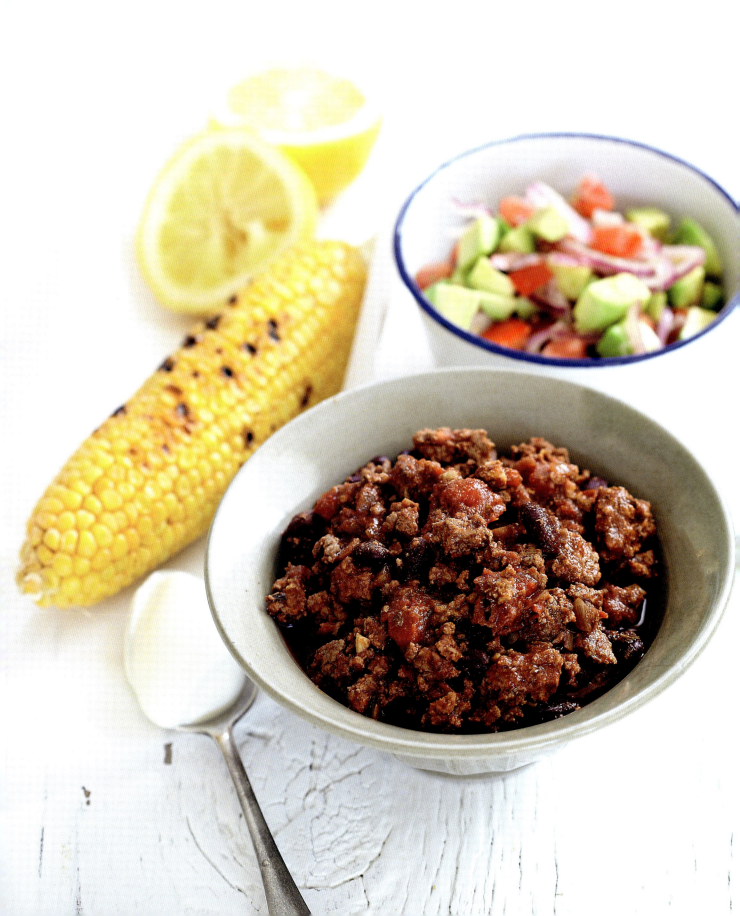

**1 SERVE =**
2 units protein
1 unit bread
¼ unit dairy
2 units vegetables
1¾ units fats

1 tablespoon olive oil
1 red (Spanish) onion, finely chopped
3 cloves garlic, chopped
1 tablespoon dried oregano
1 × 35 g packet chilli seasoning
800 g lean minced beef
1 × 400 g tin crushed tomatoes
1½ tablespoons salt-reduced tomato
    paste (puree)
1½ tablespoons red wine vinegar
2 cups (350 g) tinned red kidney
    beans, rinsed and drained
2 corn cobs
cooking oil spray
200 g reduced-fat Greek-style yoghurt
lemon halves, to serve (optional)

**AVOCADO SALAD**
1 avocado, halved, seeded and diced
2 tomatoes, seeded and chopped
½ red (Spanish) onion, finely sliced
juice of 1 lemon

# Chilli con carne with blackened corn and avocado salad

SERVES 4  PREP **15 mins**  COOK **45 mins**

**One of Mexico's most well-known exports, chilli con carne is now an Australian favourite. Packets of chilli seasoning mix are available in supermarkets, and you can also add chipotle chillies or pickled jalapenos for extra kick. Use leftover chilli con carne to make the enchiladas on page 129.**

1 Place a large heavy-based saucepan over medium–high heat. Add the oil, onion, garlic and oregano and cook for 4–5 minutes until the onion begins to soften. Stir in the seasoning mix and cook for 1 minute. Add the beef mince and cook, stirring to break up the lumps, for 5–6 minutes until the mince starts to colour. Stir in the tomatoes and tomato paste and continue to cook for 3 minutes. Add the vinegar and 3 tablespoons water, then season with salt and pepper to taste. Bring to simmering point, then reduce the heat to low, cover and simmer for 20 minutes, stirring occasionally. Add the kidney beans and cook, uncovered, for a further 10–12 minutes until the mixture has thickened and most of the liquid has evaporated (take care not to let it dry out).

2 Meanwhile, heat a barbecue or chargrill pan to high. Spray the corn lightly with cooking oil and cook, turning, for 7–8 minutes until the corn is cooked and blackened in spots. (Alternatively, steam or boil the corn until tender.) Cut each corn cob in half.

3 For the avocado salad, place all the ingredients in a bowl, season to taste with salt and pepper and toss gently to combine.

4 To serve, divide the chilli among bowls and spoon some salad alongside. Serve corn, yoghurt and lemon halves, if using, separately.

**Tip:** Make your own spice mix by combining 1 tablespoon each of ground cumin, coriander and paprika with ¾ teaspoon cayenne pepper.

# Cajun-spiced pork with braised red cabbage

SERVES 4  PREP **15 mins**  COOK **2 hours 15 mins**

3 cloves garlic, finely chopped

1 white onion, chopped, 1 tablespoon reserved for garnish

4 tablespoons pickled jalapeno chillies, drained, 1 tablespoon reserved for garnish

2 tablespoons apple cider vinegar

½ cup (180 g) tomato sauce

3 tablespoons barbecue sauce

2 tablespoons Cajun Spice Mix (see page 208)

3 teaspoons ground coriander

cooking oil spray

1 × 800 g pork shoulder, trimmed of fat, cut into 5 cm pieces

1½ cups (375 ml) Chicken Stock (see page 209)

Braised Red Cabbage with Honey and Mustard (see page 150), warm, to serve

**This is a dish for a lazy weekend. The long, slow cooking produces tender, juicy meat which just falls apart. Use any leftover pork to make the shredded pork sandwiches on page 139.**

1 Preheat the oven to 160°C.

2 Place the garlic, onion, chilli and vinegar in the bowl of a food processor and process until smooth. Stir through the sauces, spice mix and coriander and set aside.

3 Place a large heavy-based casserole over medium–high heat and spray with cooking oil. Cook the pork, in two batches if necessary, for 3–4 minutes until browned all over, then remove and set aside. Add the spicy sauce mixture to the casserole and bring to the boil. Reduce the heat to a simmer and cook, stirring occasionally, for 10–12 minutes until the onion is cooked.

4 Return the pork to the casserole, pour in the chicken stock, season to taste with salt and pepper and stir to combine. Cover, then transfer to the oven and cook for 2 hours until the pork is falling apart.

5 Using a slotted spoon, remove the pork from the sauce and transfer to a chopping board. Roughly shred with two forks, then return to the sauce and gently heat through until warm.

6 Finely chop the reserved onion and chilli and mix together.

7 Divide the warm red cabbage among plates and top with some pork and sauce. Garnish with the onion and chilli and serve.

Tip: Instead of the cabbage, you could serve this with steamed greens simply dressed with lemon juice if desired.

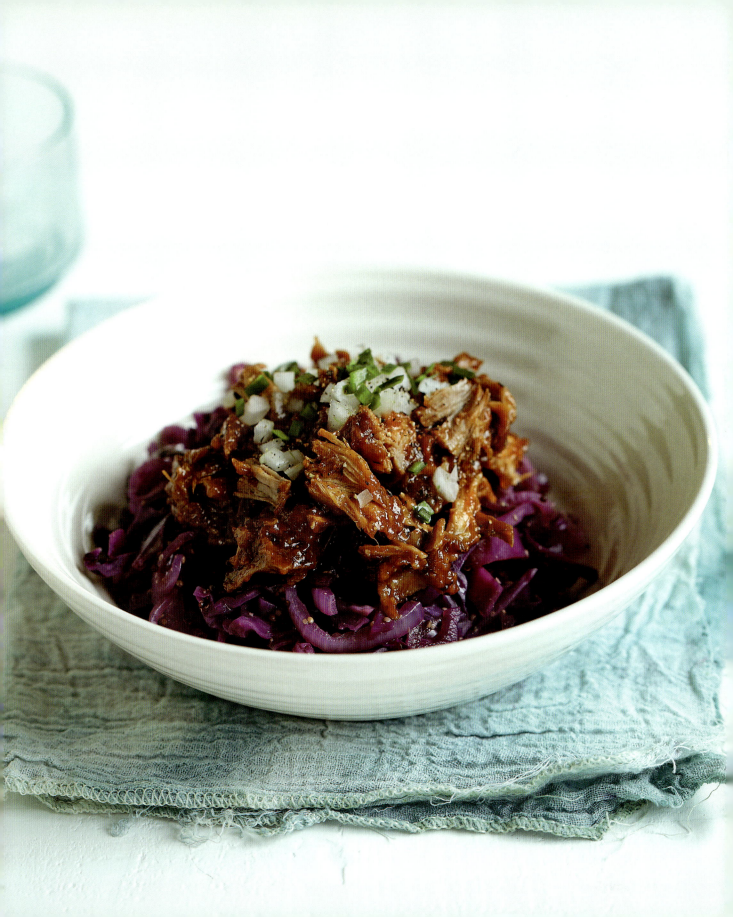

# Beef, pickled carrot and mushroom stir-fry

SERVES 4  PREP **20 mins**  COOK **15 mins**

225 g sugar snap peas

800 g beef shin, trimmed of fat and sinew, thinly sliced

1 teaspoon sesame oil

cooking oil spray

1 tablespoon peanut oil

2 cloves garlic, thinly sliced

2 tablespoons finely sliced ginger

225 g button mushrooms, quartered

6 spring onions, trimmed and finely sliced on the diagonal, a handful reserved for the garnish

1 × 410 g tin baby corn, drained, spears halved lengthways

1 cup (90 g) Pickled Carrot (see page 201) or 1 carrot, shredded

1 cup (80 g) bean sprouts

3 tablespoons oyster sauce

1 tablespoon salt-reduced soy sauce

**Beef shin is an economical cut of beef that is often used in slow-cooked braises. Here it is cooked quickly over high heat, ensuring that it remains tender and full of flavour. It's important when stir-frying not to overload the wok – cook the beef in batches to ensure it cooks evenly.**

1 Bring a saucepan of water to the boil, add the sugar snap peas and cook for 2 minutes. Drain and refresh in cold water, then drain again and set aside.

2 Place the sliced beef in a bowl, season with pepper, add the sesame oil and toss through.

3 Heat a wok or large frying pan over high heat and spray with cooking oil. Working in batches, cook the beef for 1–2 minutes until it starts to colour, then remove and set aside.

4 Add the peanut oil to the pan and heat until almost smoking. Add the garlic and ginger and cook, stirring, for 1 minute. Add the mushrooms and spring onion and cook for 2–3 minutes until the mushrooms are golden. Reduce the heat to medium–high, add the corn, carrot, peas, sprouts, oyster and soy sauces, then return the beef to the pan and cook for 2–3 minutes until the vegetables are heated through and the beef is cooked. Scatter over the reserved spring onion and serve immediately.

Tip: Serve this with steamed rice from your daily allowance.

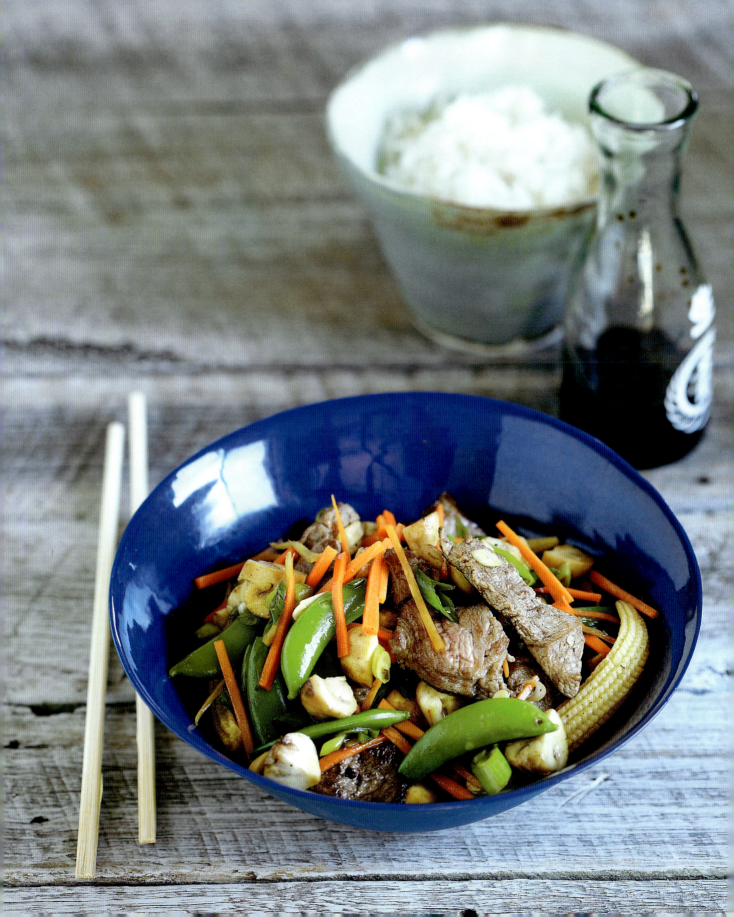

cooking oil spray

1 kg lamb forequarter chops, trimmed of fat

1 tablespoon olive oil

1 onion, chopped

2 carrots, chopped

2 sticks celery, chopped

2 tablespoons Moroccan spice mix, plus 1 teaspoon extra

½ bunch coriander, roots and stems finely chopped, leaves roughly chopped

1 × 400 g tin peeled tomatoes

2 pieces preserved lemon, rind only, rinsed and finely chopped, or finely grated zest of 1 lemon

3 cups (750 ml) Chicken Stock (see page 209)

¾ cup (160 g) French-style (puy) lentils, rinsed and drained

600 g pumpkin (squash), skin on, seeded and cut into 1.5 cm wedges

2 tablespoons Harissa (see page 205), to serve (optional)

# Moroccan-spiced lamb with lentils and roast pumpkin

SERVES 4   PREP **20 mins**   COOK **2 hours 20 mins**

**Slow-cooking lamb chops is a great alternative to cooking them on the barbecue – it adds a whole new depth of flavour. Serve the chops whole if you prefer.**

1 Place a large heavy-based stockpot over medium–high heat and spray with cooking oil. Working in batches, add the lamb chops and cook for 4–5 minutes until browned. Remove and set aside.

2 Reduce the heat to medium and add the olive oil. When hot, add the onion, carrot and celery and cook, stirring, for 7–8 minutes until the vegetables are soft. Add the Moroccan spice mix and the coriander stems and roots and cook for 2 minutes, then add the tomato, preserved lemon or lemon zest and stock. Return the lamb to the pot, season with salt and pepper to taste and bring to the boil. Reduce the heat to low and simmer for 1 hour. Add the lentils, cover with the lid and simmer for 1 hour or until the lamb and lentils are tender.

3 Meanwhile, preheat the oven to 220°C. Place the pumpkin in a single layer on a baking-paper-lined tray and spray with cooking oil. Sprinkle with the extra Moroccan spice mix, season with salt and pepper to taste and roast for 25–30 minutes until golden and tender.

4 Remove the lamb chops to a chopping board, allow to cool for 5 minutes, then strip the meat from the bones and roughly chop. Return the meat to the pot and heat over low heat until just warmed through. Stir in the chopped coriander leaves, reserving some to use as garnish.

5 To serve, spoon the lamb and lentils onto plates, arrange the pumpkin wedges to one side and garnish with the reserved chopped coriander leaves. Serve the harissa alongside, if using.

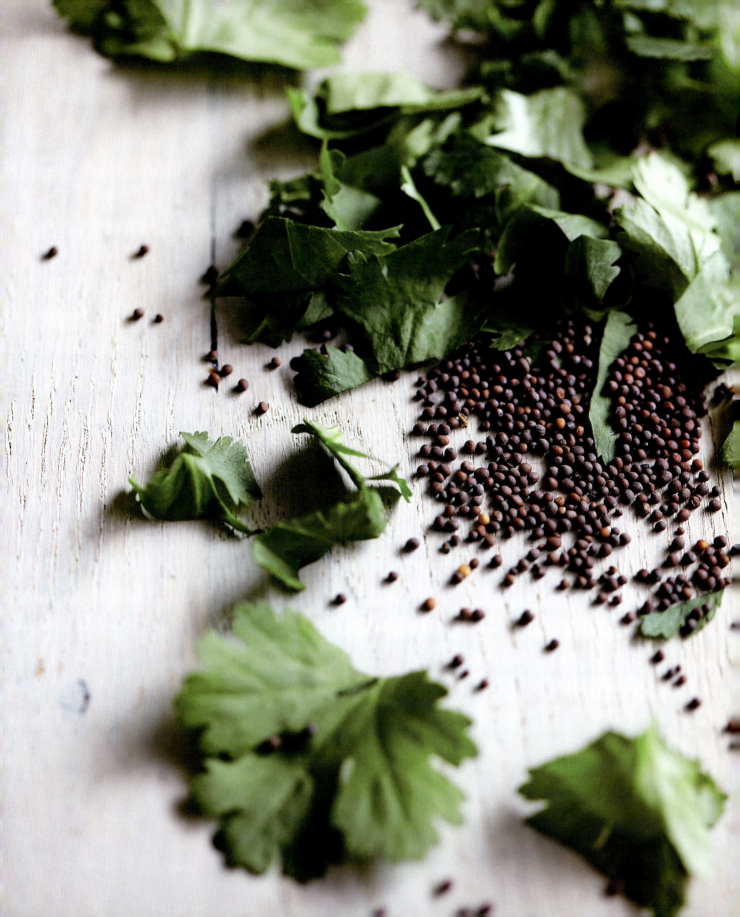

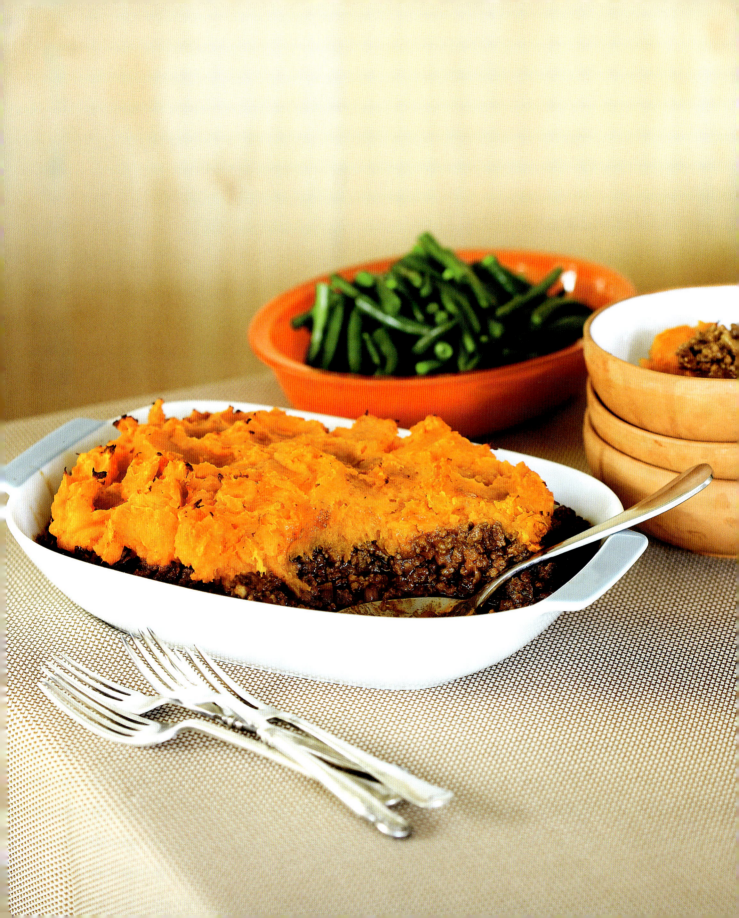

1 tablespoon olive oil

1 onion, finely chopped

3 cloves garlic, crushed

800 g lean minced lamb

1½ tablespoons ground cumin,
plus ½ teaspoon extra

1 tablespoon ground ginger

2 teaspoons sweet paprika

2 teaspoons ground cinnamon,
plus ½ teaspoon extra

2 pieces preserved lemon, rind only,
rinsed and finely chopped

½ cup (80 g) sultanas, chopped

185 ml Chicken Stock (see page 209),
plus 2 tablespoons extra

600 g pumpkin (squash), peeled,
seeded and chopped

cooking oil spray

400 g green beans, trimmed

# Middle Eastern shepherd's pie with pumpkin and green beans

SERVES 4 PREP **15 mins** COOK **1 hour**

**A new spin on an English classic, this subtly spiced version transforms the humble shepherd's pie into a dinnertime favourite. Prepare and assemble the pie in advance, then simply pop it in the oven to finish cooking.**

1 Preheat the oven to 180°C.

2 Place a large heavy-based saucepan over medium–high heat. Add the oil, onion and garlic and cook, stirring, for 4–5 minutes until the onion begins to soften. Add the lamb mince and cook, stirring to break up the lumps, for 7–8 minutes until well browned. Add the ground spices, preserved lemon and sultanas and cook for 1 minute. Add the chicken stock, season to taste with salt and pepper and stir to combine. Reduce the heat to low, cover and simmer for 10 minutes, then remove the lid and simmer for a further 2–3 minutes until most of the stock has evaporated.

3 Meanwhile, boil or steam the pumpkin until just tender. Mash together with the extra cumin, cinnamon and chicken stock until smooth.

4 Spray a 2 litre capacity ovenproof dish with cooking oil. Fill the dish with the mince mixture and spread the pumpkin mash on top. Bake for 30 minutes until the top is golden.

5 Meanwhile, boil or steam the green beans until tender.

6 To serve, cut the pie into quarters and serve with green beans alongside.

**Tip:** For an extra flavour kick, add 1½ tablespoons of a spice blend such as ras el hanout or za'atar with the other ground spices. If you're growing your own herbs, stir some chopped coriander and mint into the cooked mince.

# Malaysian beef curry with pickled cucumber

SERVES 4  PREP **15 mins**  COOK **2 hours 10 mins**

800 g chuck or blade steak, trimmed
    of fat and cut into 4 cm pieces
2 cups (500 ml) salt-reduced
    beef stock
1 tablespoon tamarind puree
400 g (3–4 individual) bok choy,
    stalks and leaves separated
    and washed
2 tablespoons desiccated coconut
1 cup (150 g) Pickled Cucumber
    (see page 201)

**MALAYSIAN CURRY PASTE**
1 onion, chopped
4 cloves garlic, chopped
3–4 small red chillies, chopped
1½ tablespoons chopped ginger
1 tablespoon peanut oil
3 teaspoons ground cumin
¼ teaspoon ground cloves
½ teaspoon ground cinnamon
½ teaspoon ground fennel seeds

**Malaysian curries are pungent, aromatic and deeply flavoured. This version includes pickled cucumber to balance the heat and richness of the beef.**

1 For the curry paste, blend the onion, garlic, chilli, ginger and oil in a food processor to a smooth paste. Stir in the ground spices and season well with pepper.

2 Heat a large heavy-based saucepan over medium–high heat. Add the spice paste and cook, stirring, for 5 minutes until fragrant. Add the beef and cook, turning to coat in the paste, for 3–4 minutes until the beef is browned. Stir in the stock, tamarind puree and 1 cup (250 ml) water and bring to the boil. Lower the heat and simmer gently, stirring occasionally, for 2 hours or until the beef is very tender. Season to taste with salt and pepper.

3 Meanwhile, steam the bok choy for 2–3 minutes until tender. Toast the coconut in a dry frying pan for a minute or two until lightly golden.

4 To serve, spoon the curry into bowls, top with pickled cucumber and scatter over the toasted coconut. Serve the steamed bok choy to the side.

**Tip:** For a quick cucumber pickle, make long ribbons by slicing unpeeled cucumber lengthways with a vegetable peeler. Lay the slices on a plate and splash with white vinegar. Leave to marinate for 20 minutes, then drain and serve.

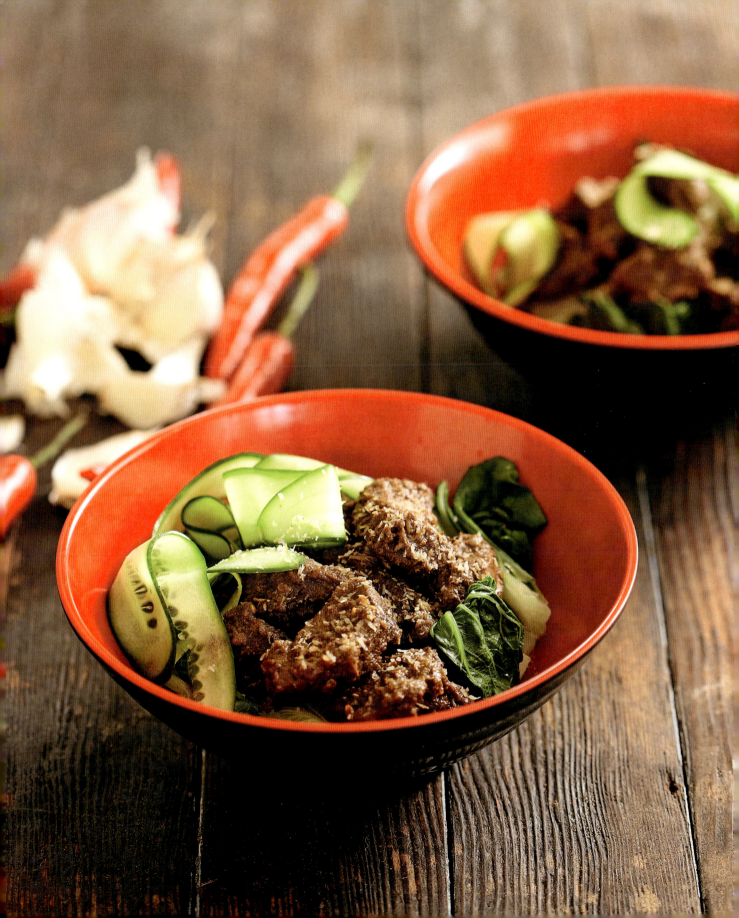

# Roast beef with beetroot, onions and chimichurri salsa

SERVES 6  PREP **15 mins, plus marinating time**  COOK **1 hour, plus resting time**

1 tablespoon dried Italian herb mix

1 teaspoon sweet paprika

¼ teaspoon chilli powder
   or cayenne pepper

2 cloves garlic, finely chopped

2 tablespoons red wine vinegar

1.2 kg beef topside roast or rib roast

1 tomato, seeded and chopped

2 brown onions, each cut into
   eight wedges

1 bunch beetroot, trimmed, peeled
   and cut into 3 cm thick wedges

Green Salad (see page 155), to serve

**MUSTARD DRESSING**

1 tablespoon extra virgin olive oil

2 tablespoons white balsamic vinegar

1 tablespoons lemon juice

2 teaspoons wholegrain mustard

**Chimichurri is an Argentinean salsa made with dried herbs, garlic and vinegar. Left to marinate, the flavour intensifies and is the perfect accompaniment to roast beef. Make extra and keep a jar in the fridge – it will last for up to 2 weeks.**

1 Combine the dried herbs, paprika, chilli powder or cayenne pepper, garlic and red wine vinegar in a bowl. Divide the mixture in half.

2 Place the beef in a shallow dish, rub half the spice mix into the beef, then cover and marinate at room temperature for 45 minutes.

3 Combine the remaining spice mix with the tomato and 2 teaspoons water in a bowl. Season to taste with salt and pepper, then set the salsa aside until ready to use.

4 Preheat the oven to 230°C. Place the beef and onion wedges in a roasting tin and season to taste with salt and pepper. Wrap the beetroot wedges in foil and place in the tin. Roast for 15 minutes, then reduce the oven temperature to 180°C and continue to roast for another 40–45 minutes for medium–rare.

5 Remove the beef from the oven, cover with foil and set aside to rest for 20 minutes. If the beetroot is tender (a skewer should pass easily through the wedges), turn the oven off but leave them inside with the onion to keep warm until ready to serve. If not, roast for another 5–10 minutes until tender.

6 For the mustard dressing, combine all the ingredients and season to taste, then toss through the green salad.

7 Thinly slice the beef, then stir in 3 teaspoons of the resting juices to the salsa. Divide the beef and vegetables between plates. Serve with the salsa and green salad to the side.

**Tip:** Don't be tempted to skip the resting step: the meat will not be as tender if eaten straight away.

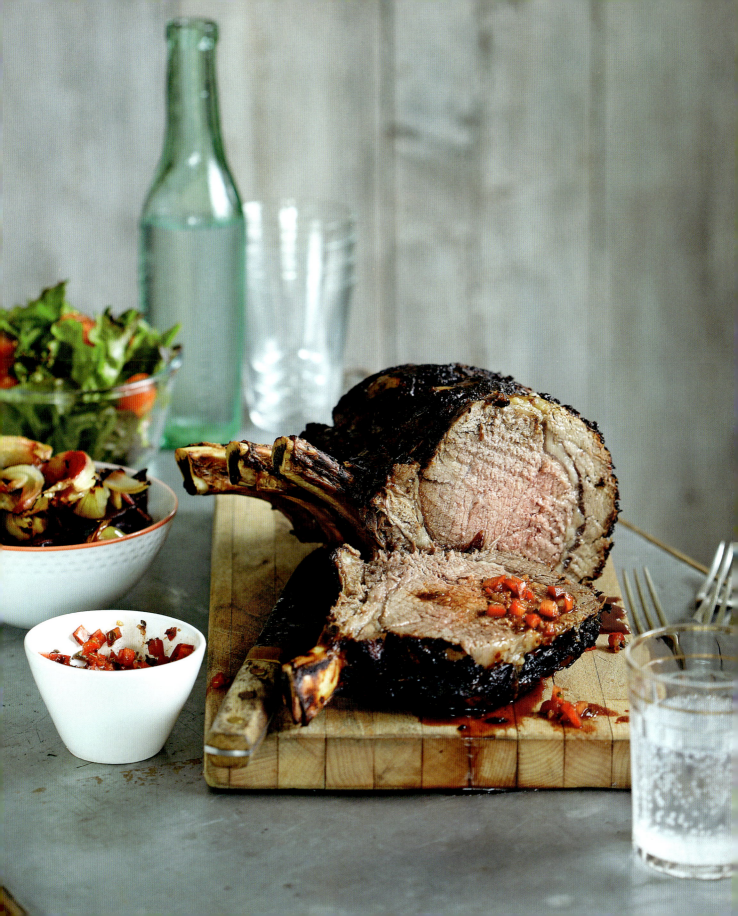

# Paprika pork chops with braised silverbeet

SERVES 4  PREP **15 mins, plus marinating time**  COOK **30 mins**

2 teaspoons smoked paprika

1 teaspoon sweet paprika

1 teaspoon ground coriander

2 cloves garlic, finely chopped

finely grated zest and juice of 1 lemon

800 g pork chops or cutlets,
   trimmed of fat

cooking oil spray

lemon wedges, to serve

**BRAISED SILVERBEET**

1 tablespoon olive oil

1 red (Spanish) onion, finely chopped

2 cloves garlic, sliced

¼–½ teaspoon chilli flakes

600 g (2 bunches) silverbeet
   (Swiss chard), well washed,
   stems removed and finely
   chopped, leaves shredded

4 tablespoons Chicken Stock
   (see page 209) or water

1½ tablespoons red wine vinegar

**Silverbeet is economical, packed full of nutrients and goes beautifully with pork, chicken or red meat. The stems are often thrown away but they are delicious – just finely chop them and cook them for a bit longer than the leaves.**

1 Place the smoked and sweet paprika, coriander, garlic and lemon zest and juice in a small bowl and mix together. Place the pork in a shallow dish, season to taste with salt and pepper and spoon over the marinade. Toss to coat and set aside for 30–60 minutes to marinate.

2 For the braised silverbeet, place a large saucepan over medium–high heat. Add the olive oil, onion, garlic, chilli and silverbeet stems and cook for 3–4 minutes until the onion begins to soften. Stir in the silverbeet leaves and the stock or water, then reduce the heat to low and cook, covered, for 20–25 minutes until the leaves are soft and have turned a dark green colour. Stir through the vinegar and season with salt and pepper to taste.

3 Meanwhile, heat a barbecue or chargrill pan to high and spray with cooking oil. Cook the pork for 5–6 minutes on each side until cooked. Cover and rest for 5 minutes.

4 To serve, divide the silverbeet among four plates, top each with a pork chop and serve with lemon wedges.

Tip: For some extra vegetable units, serve this with Honey-roasted Carrots with Cumin and Caraway (see page 146).

cooking oil spray
800 g chuck or blade steak, trimmed
   of fat and cut into 3 cm pieces
1 tablespoon olive oil
350 g golden shallots (about 12)
   or small pickling onions, peeled
2 carrots, roughly chopped
3 cloves garlic, chopped
3 sprigs rosemary, chopped or
   1 tablespoon dried rosemary
3 sprigs thyme or 2 teaspoons
   dried thyme
500 ml Slow-roasted Tomato Sauce
   (see page 198) or salt-reduced
   tomato passata
1 cup (250 ml) salt-reduced
   beef stock or water
finely grated zest and juice of 1 lemon
300 g button mushrooms, halved
4 zucchinis (courgettes),
   halved lengthways
Parsnip and Cauliflower Puree (see
   page 149), to serve (optional)

# Braised beef, rosemary and mushroom casserole

SERVES 4   PREP **20 mins**   COOK **2 hours 20 mins**

**Chuck steak is perfect for braising as it becomes meltingly soft with long, slow cooking. For a deeper flavour, splash in some red wine when adding the herbs, and cook until reduced by half, before returning the beef to the pan. Serve with parsnip and cauliflower puree to boost your vegetable intake (this adds 2 units).**

1 Place a large flameproof casserole over medium–high heat and spray with cooking oil. Add the beef in two batches and cook for 4–5 minutes until browned on all sides, then remove and set aside.

2 Reduce the heat to medium and add the olive oil. Add the shallots or onions and carrot and cook for 5–6 minutes until the shallots are golden. Add the garlic, rosemary and thyme and cook for 2 minutes. Return the beef to the pan, along with the tomato sauce or passata, stock or water and lemon zest. Season to taste with salt and pepper, then stir to combine and bring to the boil. Cover, reduce the heat to low and simmer for 1 hour 30 minutes. Add the mushrooms, then simmer uncovered for another 20–30 minutes until the beef and mushrooms are tender.

3 Meanwhile, steam the zucchini for 8–10 minutes until tender. Transfer to a bowl, squeeze over the lemon juice and season with pepper.

4 Spoon the casserole into shallow bowls and serve with the zucchini to the side. Serve with cauliflower and parsnip puree if desired.

**Tip:** If you like a thicker sauce, at the end of the cooking time mix 1 tablespoon flour with 3 tablespoons of the braising liquid to make a smooth paste, then stir the paste through the sauce and cook until thickened.

# Spiced lamb chops with sauteed mustard cabbage

SERVES 4  PREP **20 mins**  COOK **1 hour 35 mins**

cooking oil spray

1 kg (8 chops) lamb loin chops, trimmed of fat

2 teaspoons vegetable oil

1 onion, finely chopped

1 tablespoon finely grated ginger

4 cloves garlic, crushed

½ bunch coriander, roots and stems finely chopped, leaves chopped and reserved

3 teaspoons ground coriander

2 teaspoons ground cumin

1 teaspoon cayenne pepper

125 g reduced-fat Greek-style yoghurt

SAUTEED MUSTARD CABBAGE

2 teaspoons vegetable oil

2 teaspoons brown mustard seeds

¼ white cabbage (300 g), finely shredded

2 carrots, grated

1 teaspoon ground turmeric

2 tablespoons reduced-fat plain yoghurt

**Cooking lamb in yoghurt helps to tenderise and flavour the meat, and results in a rich and creamy sauce that is low in fat.**

1 Place a large heavy-based casserole over medium–high heat and spray with cooking oil. Cook the chops, in two batches if necessary, for 4–5 minutes until browned, then remove from the pan and set aside.

2 Heat the oil in the casserole, then add the onion and cook for 7–8 minutes until golden. Add the ginger, garlic and coriander roots and stems and cook for 1 minute. Add the ground spices and cook, stirring, for 1 minute. Whisk the yoghurt with 1 cup (250 ml) water until combined, then add to the casserole, season to taste with salt and pepper and stir well to combine. Return the chops and any juices to the pan and bring to the boil. Reduce the heat to low, cover and simmer for 1 hour 15 minutes, stirring gently every 10 minutes or so, until the chops are very tender. Stir through the chopped coriander, reserving some to use as a garnish.

3 Meanwhile, for the sauteed cabbage, heat the oil in a medium-sized saucepan over medium–high heat. Add the mustard seeds and cook until they begin to pop. Add the cabbage and cook, stirring, for 2 minutes. Add the carrot and turmeric, season to taste with salt and pepper and stir well to coat in the spices. Add 2 tablespoons water, cover and cook for 10 minutes, stirring now and then, until the cabbage is tender. If the mixture becomes dry, add another tablespoon of water. Stir through the yoghurt.

4 To serve, divide the cabbage and chops among four plates. Drizzle over the sauce and scatter with the reserved coriander leaves.

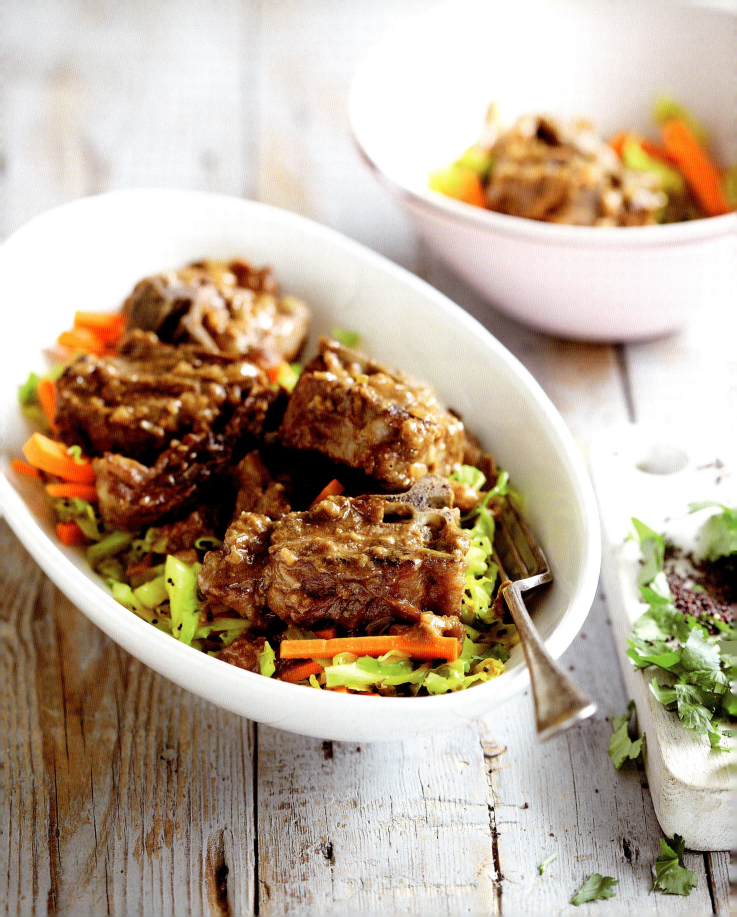

2 tomatoes
2 bunches spinach,
   washed and trimmed
cooking oil spray
1 × 800 g lamb shoulder, trimmed
   of fat and cut into 3 cm pieces
1 tablespoon vegetable oil
1 onion, finely chopped
4 cloves garlic, crushed
1 tablespoon finely grated ginger
2 tablespoons Madras Curry Powder
   (see page 208)
3 teaspoons Garam Masala
   (see page 208)
½ cup (140 g) reduced-fat
   Greek-style yoghurt
1 head cauliflower, cut into
   medium-sized florets
steamed basmati rice (optional),
   to serve

# Lamb and spinach curry with roast cauliflower

SERVES 4  PREP **20 mins**  COOK **2 hours 25 mins**

**This is a mild northern Indian curry featuring garam masala, an aromatic spice blend used widely in Indian cuisine. Serving this curry with ⅓ cup (65 g) steamed basmati rice per person will add 1 bread unit per serve.**

1  Cut a cross in the base of each tomato. Bring a saucepan of water to the boil, then remove the pan from the heat. Place the tomatoes in the water for 30 seconds, then remove with a slotted spoon. When cool enough to handle, peel off their skins and chop the flesh. Set aside.

2  Cook the spinach in a large saucepan of boiling water for 1–2 minutes until wilted. Drain well, finely chop and set aside.

3  Place a large heavy-based saucepan over medium–high heat. Spray with cooking oil and fry the lamb, in two batches, for 4–5 minutes until well browned, then remove and set aside.

4  Add the oil, onion, garlic and ginger to the pan and fry for 3–4 minutes until the onion begins to soften. Add the curry powder and 2 teaspoons of the garam masala and cook for 1 minute, stirring to prevent the spices from burning. Add the chopped tomato and cook for about 5 minutes until the tomato has broken down. Add the yoghurt, stir well to combine, then add 1¼ cups (310 ml) water. Stir in the spinach, return the lamb to the pan, then season to taste with salt and pepper and bring to the boil. Reduce the heat to low, cover and simmer for 1½–2 hours, stirring occasionally, until the lamb is tender. If the mixture becomes dry, add 2–3 tablespoons water.

5  Meanwhile, preheat the oven to 220°C. Arrange the cauliflower on two baking-paper-lined trays and spray with cooking oil. Sprinkle over the remaining garam masala and roast for 20–25 minutes until golden.

6  Serve the curry with the roast cauliflower alongside, and steamed basmati rice if desired.

**Tip:** If you don't have any fresh spinach, use 125 g frozen spinach, thawed following the instructions on the packet.

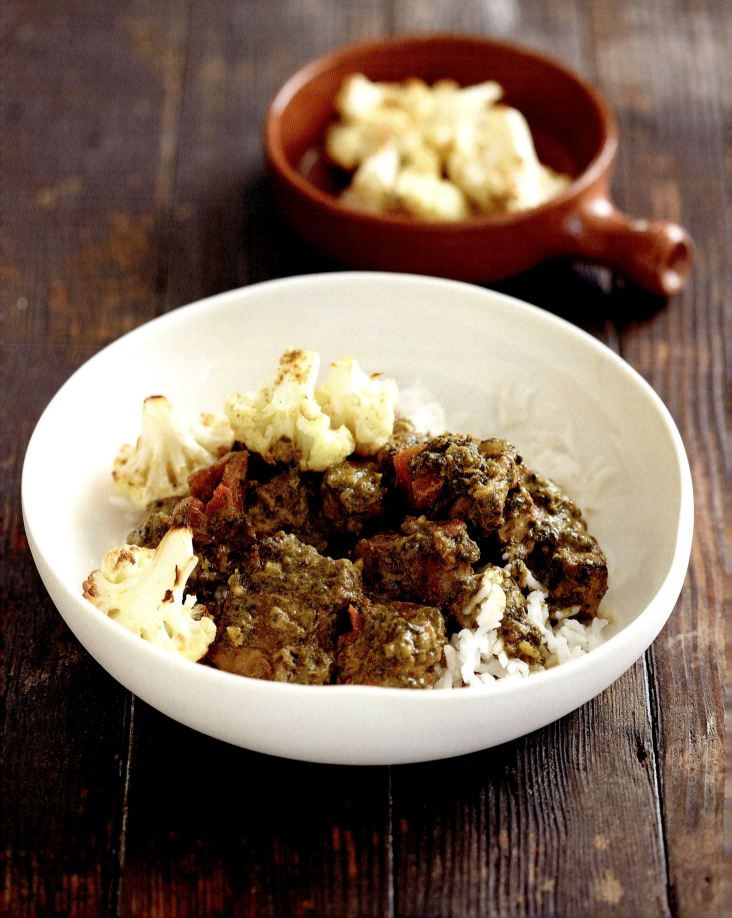

2 units protein
¼ unit fruit
2½ units vegetables

# Spiced pork meatballs with Asian slaw

SERVES 4  PREP **25 mins**  COOK **8 mins**

800 g lean minced pork
1 carrot, grated
4 spring onions, trimmed and
    finely sliced
1–2 long red chillies, seeded
    and finely chopped
1 tablespoon finely chopped ginger
1 stalk lemongrass, trimmed and
    finely chopped
2 teaspoons ground coriander
2 tablespoons fish sauce
cooking oil spray

**ASIAN SLAW**
¼ white cabbage (300 g),
    finely shredded
1 green apple, cut into
    thin matchsticks
2 large carrots, cut into thin
    matchsticks or grated
3 spring onions, trimmed and
    finely sliced
1 long red chilli (optional), seeded
    and finely sliced
1 quantity Nam Jim Dressing (see
    page 206)

**Perfect for lunch or dinner, these spiced meatballs are very versatile. Make more than you need and use them in the spiced pork salad recipe on page 134.**

1 In a bowl, combine the pork mince, carrot, spring onion, chilli, ginger, lemongrass and ground coriander. Mix together with your hands for 3–4 minutes until well combined and sticky. Add the fish sauce, season with white pepper, then mix until combined. Using wet hands, roll the mixture into walnut-sized balls.

2 Preheat the oven grill to high and place the meatballs on a baking-paper-lined tray. Spray with cooking oil and grill for 7–8 minutes, turning regularly, until golden and cooked through.

3 To make the slaw, combine the ingredients in a large bowl.

4 Add the grilled meatballs to the slaw, toss through gently and serve.

**Tip:** Add a small handful of chopped mint or coriander from your herb garden to the salad. Skewer the meatballs and cook on the barbecue for a smoky flavour.

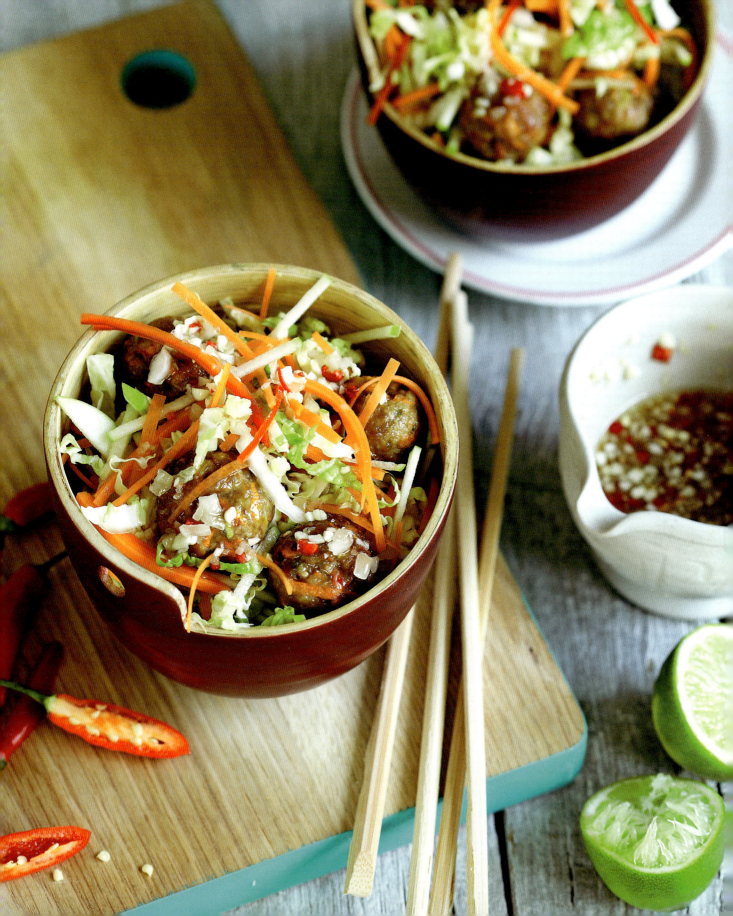

# Braised lamb shoulder with roast fennel

SERVES 4  PREP **25 mins**  COOK **2 hours 15 mins**

cooking oil spray
1 × 800 g lamb shoulder, trimmed
    of fat and cut into 3 cm pieces
1 tablespoon olive oil
1 onion, finely chopped
3 cloves garlic, finely chopped
1 tablespoon fennel seeds
1 tablespoon thyme leaves or
    2 teaspoons dried thyme
2 tablespoons salt-reduced tomato
    paste (puree)
3 teaspoons sweet paprika
1½ cups (375 ml) Chicken Stock
    (see page 209)
2 large bulbs fennel, trimmed, each
    cut into six wedges, fronds reserved
Parsnip and Cauliflower Puree
    (see page 149), warmed, to serve

**Lamb shoulder is an economical cut of meat perfect for braising as it won't dry out with long cooking. Make more than you need and use the leftovers to make a fattoush salad (see page 133) or lamb souvlakis (see page 138).**

1 Heat a large heavy-based saucepan over medium–high heat and spray with cooking oil. Cook the lamb, in batches if necessary, until browned all over. Remove from the pan and set aside.

2 Reduce the heat to medium and add the olive oil, onion, garlic, fennel seeds and thyme. Cook for 3–4 minutes until the onion begins to soften. Return the lamb to the pan, along with the tomato paste, paprika and chicken stock. Stir to combine and season lightly with salt and pepper. Bring to the boil, then reduce the heat to as low as possible, cover and simmer gently for 1½–2 hours until the meat is very tender and almost falling apart.

3 Meanwhile, preheat the oven to 200°C and line a baking tray with baking paper.

4 Place the fennel on the prepared tray, spray with cooking oil and season to taste with salt and pepper. Roast for 20–25 minutes until golden and tender.

5 To serve, spoon the puree into bowls and top with the braised lamb. Garnish with the reserved fennel fronds. Serve the roast fennel alongside.

**Tip:** Try adding fresh rosemary, sage or tarragon from your herb garden for variety.

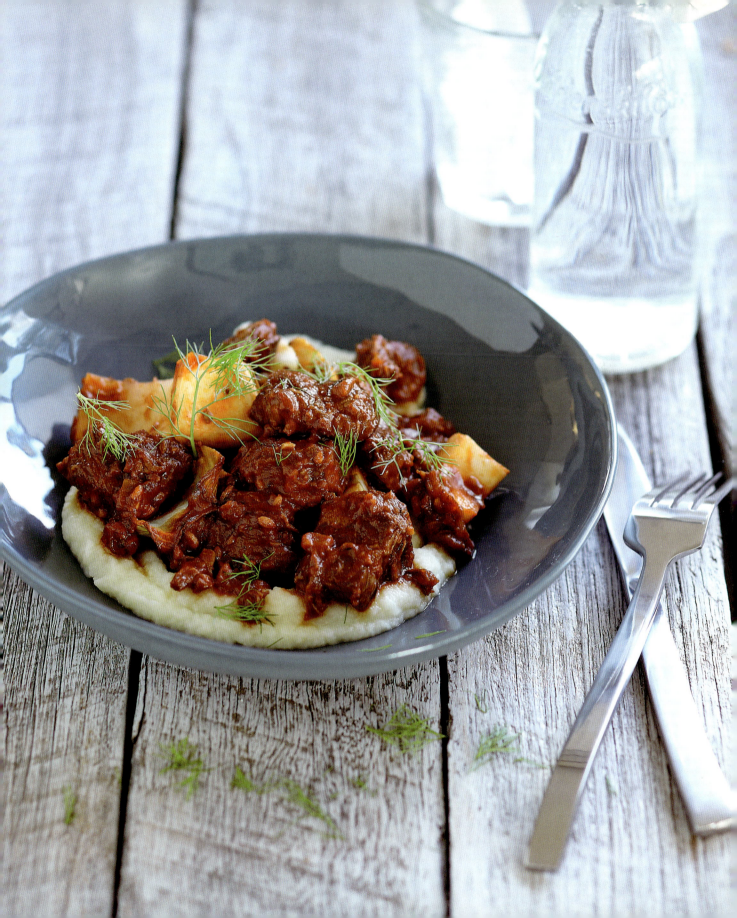

# CHICKEN
# & FISH

800 g skinless chicken thigh fillets,
    trimmed of fat, halved
3 teaspoons ground turmeric
cooking oil spray
1 tablespoon peanut or vegetable oil
2 teaspoons yellow mustard seeds
1 red (Spanish) onion, finely diced
2 long red chillies, finely sliced
1½ tablespoons finely chopped ginger
1 cinnamon stick
5 cloves
1¼ cups (310 ml) Chicken Stock
    (see page 209)
finely grated zest of 1 lemon
juice of 2 lemons
2 tablespoons sultanas
2 bunches Chinese broccoli (gai lan),
    trimmed and cut into 3 cm lengths

# Zingy lemon chicken

SERVES 4  PREP **15 mins**  COOK **25 mins**

**A fresh approach to sweet and sour chicken, this dish is zesty, fragrant and packed with flavour. Serve this with any steamed vegetables you like: try carrot, cauliflower, broccoli, snowpeas or green beans.**

1 Dust the chicken pieces all over with 2 teaspoons of the turmeric. Place a large frying pan over medium–high heat and spray with cooking oil. Working in batches, cook the chicken for 2–3 minutes until browned on all sides. Remove the chicken and set aside.

2 In the same pan, add the peanut or vegetable oil and mustard seeds and cook until the seeds begin to pop, then add the onion, chilli and ginger and cook for 2 minutes until fragrant. Add the cinnamon stick, cloves and remaining turmeric and cook for 1 minute more. Add the stock, lemon zest and juice and the sultanas and bring to the boil. Season to taste with salt and pepper, then return the chicken to the pan. Stir to combine, then reduce the heat to low and simmer, covered, for 10–12 minutes until the chicken is cooked through. Transfer the chicken to a plate with a slotted spoon and cover to keep warm. Increase the heat to high and boil the sauce, uncovered, for 2–3 minutes until thickened and reduced.

3 Meanwhile, steam or boil the Chinese broccoli for 3–4 minutes until just tender, then drain.

4 To serve, divide the Chinese broccoli among four plates, top with the chicken and spoon over the sauce.

Tip: For some added sweetness, add 1 finely chopped red capsicum along with the spices and cook for 2 minutes. You could use fish or prawns instead of chicken (just adjust the cooking time accordingly).

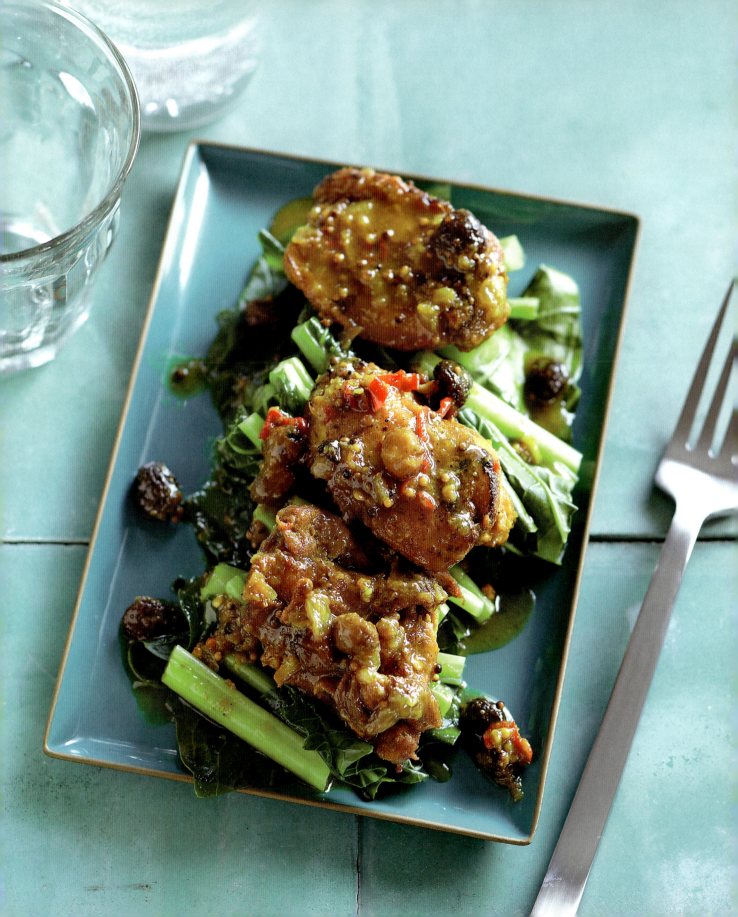

4 × 200 g snapper fillets, skin-on
   and bones removed
3 tablespoons fish sauce
4 red shallots or ½ small red
   (Spanish) onion, chopped
1 stalk lemongrass, white part only,
   finely chopped
1½ tablespoons Thai Green Curry
   Paste (see page 205) or ready-made
   Thai green curry paste
1 teaspoon ground coriander
½ teaspoon ground turmeric
1¼ cups (310 ml) reduced-fat
   coconut-flavoured evaporated milk
2 teaspoons palm or brown sugar
cooking oil spray
1 bunch baby bok choy, washed
   and halved
lime wedges, to serve (optional)

# Simple Thai green fish curry

SERVES 4  PREP **15 mins**  COOK **15 mins**

**The spiciest of the Thai curry varieties, this green curry is full-flavoured, low in fat and works well with any kind of seafood or chicken. Be careful not to allow the evaporated milk to boil as it can curdle easily.**

1 Rub the fish fillets all over with 1 tablespoon of the fish sauce and set aside.

2 In a food processor, blend the shallot or onion and lemongrass until combined (or you can do this using a mortar and pestle). Add the green curry paste, coriander and turmeric, season with pepper and blend again until smooth.

3 Bring the evaporated milk to simmering point in a small saucepan (being careful not to let it boil), then add the sugar and remaining fish sauce and stir to combine. Reduce the heat, then take 3 tablespoons of the hot milk mixture and add it to the paste. Mix well to combine, then add back to the pan. Return to simmering point and cook, stirring, for 4–5 minutes until aromatic. Season to taste with salt and pepper.

4 Heat a large frying pan over high heat until very hot. Pat the fish dry and spray all over with cooking oil, then season with salt and pepper to taste. Cook the fish, skin-side down, in the hot pan for 3–4 minutes, then turn and cook for 1–2 minutes or until cooked through (the cooking time will vary depending on the thickness of the fish).

5 Meanwhile, steam or boil the bok choy for 2–3 minutes until just tender, then drain.

6 Divide the bok choy among plates, top with a piece of fish and spoon over the sauce. Serve with lime wedges if desired.

**Tip:** For a spicier curry, add 2–3 chopped small green chillies to the paste along with the shallot or onion.

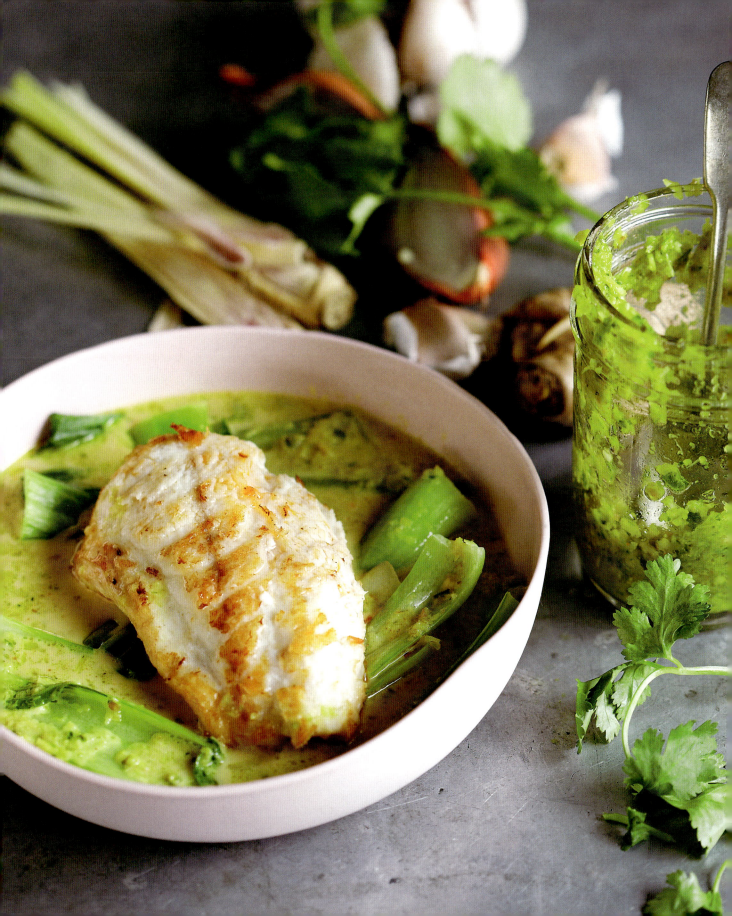

1 iceberg lettuce, cored
lime wedges and finely sliced
   red chilli, to serve

**PORK FILLING**
1 tablespoon peanut oil
4 cloves garlic, finely chopped
2 long red chillies, seeded and
   finely sliced
2 tablespoons finely chopped ginger
½ bunch coriander, stems and roots
   finely chopped, leaves reserved
800 g lean minced pork
150 g green beans, trimmed and
   finely sliced
1 carrot, cut into thin matchsticks
100 g mushrooms, sliced
2½ tablespoons fish sauce
2 tablespoons lime or lemon juice
2 teaspoons palm or brown sugar
2 cups (160 g) bean sprouts

# Thai-style san choi bao

SERVES 4  PREP **20 mins, plus soaking time**  COOK **10 mins**

**This classic Chinese dish served in lettuce cups is given a Thai twist with the addition of fish sauce and lime juice. Soaking the whole lettuce in cold water helps the leaves to separate and come away without tearing. Use a pair of scissors to trim each lettuce cup to an even size. If you like, make extra pork filling to use in the spring roll recipe on page 134.**

1 Soak the lettuce in a large bowl of cold water for 30 minutes. Gently separate the leaves, drain and refrigerate until ready to use.

2 For the pork filling, heat a large wok or frying pan over high heat and add the peanut oil. When hot, add the garlic, chilli, ginger and coriander stems and roots and stir-fry for 1 minute until fragrant. Add the pork mince and cook, stirring and breaking up the lumps with a wooden spoon, for 2–3 minutes until the mince changes colour. Add the green beans, carrot and mushroom and continue to stir-fry for 3–4 minutes until the vegetables are tender and the pork is cooked. Stir through the fish sauce, lime or lemon juice and sugar, then season lightly with salt and pepper and toss to combine.

3 Remove the wok from the heat and toss through the bean sprouts and coriander leaves, reserving a small amount to use as garnish.

4 To serve, divide the pork filling among the lettuce cups and garnish with the remaining bean sprouts and coriander. Offer lime wedges and sliced chilli to the side.

**Tip:** For extra crunch, add 4 tablespoons chopped Pickled Radish (see page 201) or 4 tablespoons chopped water chestnuts along with the bean sprouts at the end.

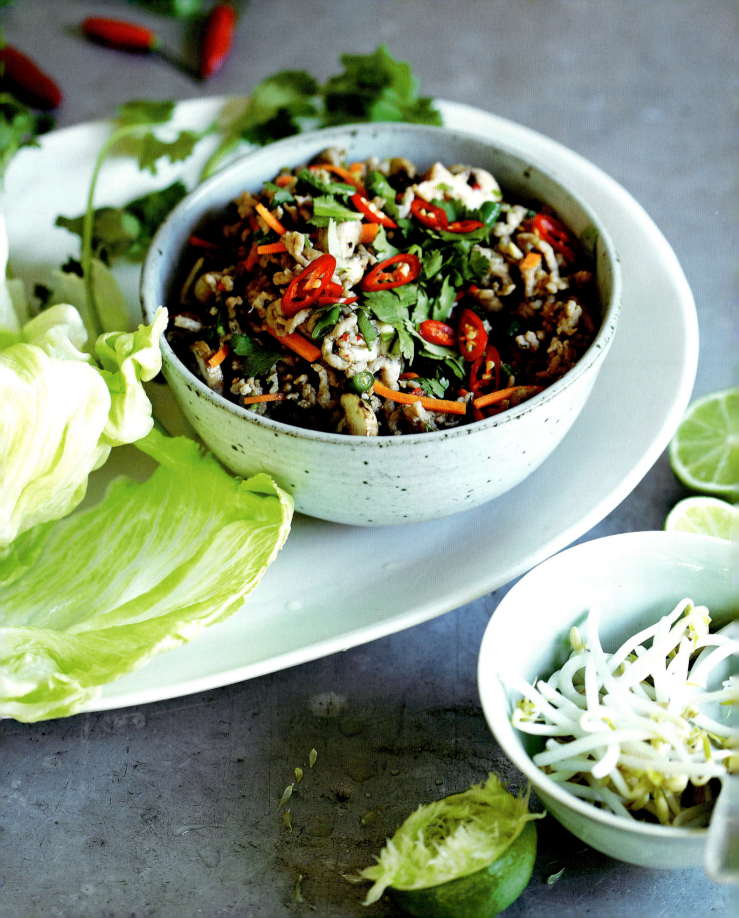

# Pan-fried fish with ginger and miso broth

SERVES 4  PREP **15 mins**  COOK **20 mins**

2 teaspoons sesame seeds

3 cups (750 ml) Chicken Stock (see
page 209) or salt-reduced fish stock

3 spring onions, trimmed, white part
sliced, green part finely sliced on
the diagonal

2 tablespoons finely chopped ginger

1½ tablespoons mirin

½ teaspoon sesame oil

2 tablespoons white miso paste

2 bunches asparagus, trimmed,
cut into 5 cm lengths

1 cup (120 g) frozen peas

1 × 410 g tin baby corn, drained,
halved lengthways

cooking oil spray

800 g white fish fillets (such as
blue-eye, ling or snapper), skin
and bones removed

1 cup (80 g) bean sprouts

**This delicate and fragrant broth, lightly scented with ginger and sesame oil, teams beautifully with firm white fish such as blue-eye, ling or snapper.**

1  Place the sesame seeds in a small frying pan over medium heat and toast, stirring, for 2–3 minutes until lightly golden.

2  Place the stock, the white part of the spring onion, ginger, mirin and sesame oil in a saucepan and bring to the boil. Reduce the heat and simmer, covered, for 10 minutes. Place the miso paste in a bowl. Take ½ cup (125 ml) hot stock and add to the miso paste, mixing until smooth. Repeat with another ½ cup (125 ml) stock, then return the miso mixture to the saucepan. Bring to simmering point (being careful not to let it boil), then add the asparagus. Cook for 2 minutes, then add the peas and corn and cook for a further 2 minutes until the asparagus is tender. Remove from the heat and season with white pepper.

3  Meanwhile, place a large non-stick frying pan over high heat and spray with cooking oil. Season the fish with salt and pepper and cook, skin-side down, for 3 minutes, then turn and cook for 1–1½ minutes on the other side until cooked through (the cooking time will vary depending on the thickness of the fish).

4  To serve, divide the vegetables among four shallow bowls and top each with a fillet of fish. Pour over the broth, then garnish with the bean sprouts, sesame seeds and reserved spring onion.

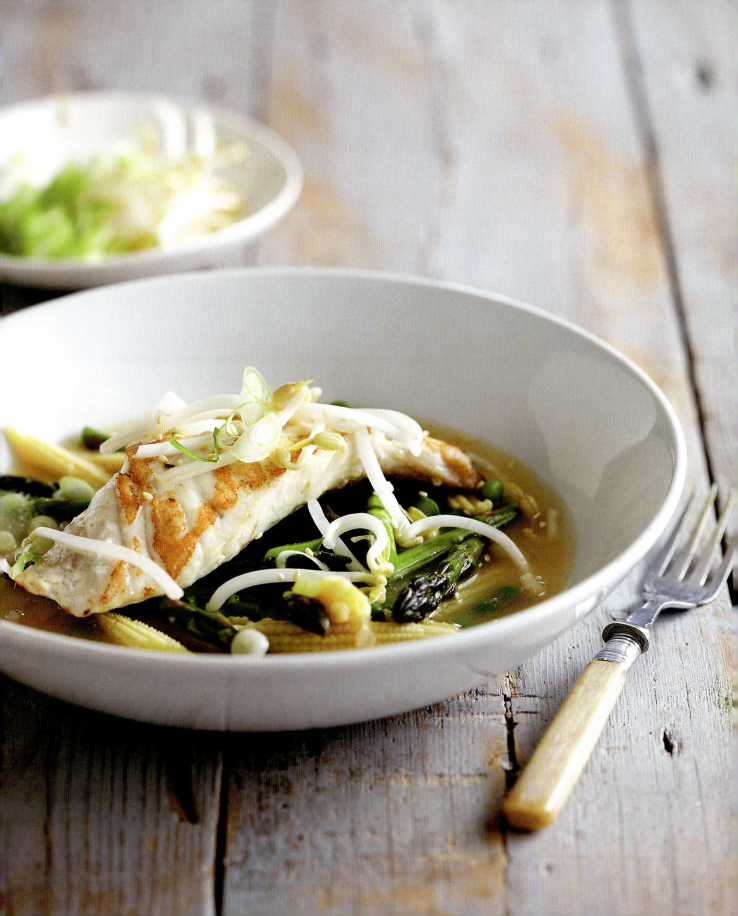

1 tablespoon olive oil
1 small onion, finely chopped
2 carrots, chopped
2 sticks celery, chopped
2 cloves garlic, finely chopped
2 bay leaves
1.25 litres Chicken Stock
   (see page 209)
800 g skinless chicken thigh fillets,
   trimmed of fat
4 tablespoons long-grain rice
2 eggs
2 tablespoons lemon juice
1 tablespoon finely chopped
   flat-leaf parsley

# Greek garlic and lemon soup with rice and chicken

SERVES 4  PREP **10 mins**  COOK **40 mins, plus cooling time**

**This modern version of a Greek classic is hearty, tangy and utterly satisfying.**

1 Place a large stockpot over medium heat. Add the olive oil, onion, carrot and celery and cook for 7–8 minutes until the vegetables are very soft but not coloured. Add the garlic and bay leaves and cook for 2 minutes before adding the stock and 2 cups (500 ml) water. Bring to the boil, then reduce the heat and simmer for 10 minutes. Add the chicken, return to simmering point and cook for 8 minutes. Turn off the heat and leave the chicken to cool in the stock for 15 minutes. Remove the chicken with a slotted spoon and, when cool enough to handle, finely shred.

2 Return the soup to the boil, add the rice and cook for 10 minutes until the rice is tender. Turn off the heat, remove the bay leaves and leave to soup to stand for 2 minutes.

3 In a small bowl, whisk the eggs until frothy, then whisk in the lemon juice. Take 1 cup (250 ml) of the hot soup from the pot and whisk it into the egg and lemon mixture until well combined. Pour the mixture back into the pot, whisking continuously until thickened. Place the soup over low heat and simmer for 2 minutes to heat through (be careful not to let it boil). Season to taste with salt and pepper and stir through the parsley just before serving.

**Tip:** Leaving the chicken to cool in the stock helps keep the flesh tender and juicy.

**1 SERVE =**
2 units protein
2½ units vegetables
1 unit fats

# Chicken baked in a parcel with mushrooms and cherry tomatoes

SERVES 4  PREP **15 mins, plus marinating time** COOK **30 mins**

800 g skinless chicken thigh cutlets,
　trimmed of fat
3 cloves garlic, thinly sliced
2 teaspoons extra virgin olive oil
1 teaspoon dried oregano
1 teaspoon fennel seeds
1 × 250 g punnet cherry tomatoes,
　quartered or halved
250–350 g field mushrooms,
　thickly sliced
1 lemon, peeled and thinly sliced
　into rounds
½ cup (125 ml) Chicken Stock
　(see page 209) or white wine
Sumac-spiced Broccoli and Peas
　(see page 152), to serve

**Baking in a parcel is a mess-free way to maximise flavour by locking in all the moisture normally lost during cooking. Experiment using different spices or fresh herbs.**

1 Preheat the oven to 200°C.

2 In a bowl, combine the chicken, garlic, olive oil, oregano, fennel seeds and cherry tomatoes and season to taste with salt and pepper. Cover and leave to marinate for 30–60 minutes.

3 Cut four lengths of foil about 40 cm long and place two pieces on top of each other. Fold in three sides, leaving one long side open. Repeat with remaining foil, then place both parcels on a large baking tray. Divide the mushrooms between the foil parcels, then top each with half the chicken mixture and lemon slices. Pour half the stock into each parcel, then fold the open end over a few times to seal tightly. Bake for 30 minutes. Remove from the oven and leave to stand for 3 minutes.

4 Carefully break open the parcels, divide the chicken mixture among four plates and serve with the broccoli and peas.

# Chicken tikka with turmeric-braised green beans

SERVES 4   PREP **15 mins, plus marinating time**   COOK **30 mins**

800 g skinless chicken thigh fillets,
    trimmed of fat
1 tablespoon vegetable oil
½ teaspoon ground turmeric
600 g green beans, trimmed
    and halved
juice of ½ lemon
small handful roughly chopped
    coriander leaves
1 teaspoon Garam Masala
    (see page 208)
lemon wedges, to serve

**TIKKA CURRY PASTE**
6 cloves garlic, chopped
2 tablespoons chopped ginger
1–2 small red chillies, chopped
¼ bunch coriander, stems and
    roots chopped
juice of 1 lemon
1 tablespoon Garam Masala
    (see page 208)
1 teaspoon sweet paprika
3 tablespoons reduced-fat
    Greek-style yoghurt

**One of India's most recognisable dishes, these spicy, yoghurt-marinated chicken pieces are great to serve for a dinner party. Use any leftovers to make the chicken tikka wraps on page 137.**

1 Place the chicken pieces in a large shallow bowl.

2 For the curry paste, blend the garlic, ginger, chillies, coriander stems and roots and the lemon juice together to form a smooth paste. Reserve 1 tablespoon of the mixture to flavour the green beans, and to the remaining paste, add the garam masala, paprika and yoghurt. Mix well, season to taste with salt and pepper, then spoon over the chicken pieces. Turn to coat, then cover and marinate for 2 hours or overnight in the fridge.

3 Preheat the oven to 200°C. Arrange the chicken pieces on a rack positioned over a roasting tin, and roast for 20–25 minutes until the chicken is cooked through and the edges have started to darken.

4 Meanwhile, place a medium-sized saucepan over medium heat, add the oil and reserved paste and cook, stirring, for 2 minutes. Add the turmeric and green beans and cook, stirring, for 1 minute until the beans are coated in the spice mix. Add the lemon juice and 1 tablespoon of warm water, then reduce the heat to low, cover and cook for 20–25 minutes until the beans are tender. Season with salt and pepper, then toss through the chopped coriander.

5 To serve, divide the beans among plates and sprinkle over 1 teaspoon garam masala. Top with the chicken pieces and serve with lemon wedges.

Tip: For a chargrilled flavour, cook the chicken under a preheated grill or on the barbecue – it should take 8–10 minutes, but check the chicken is cooked through before serving.

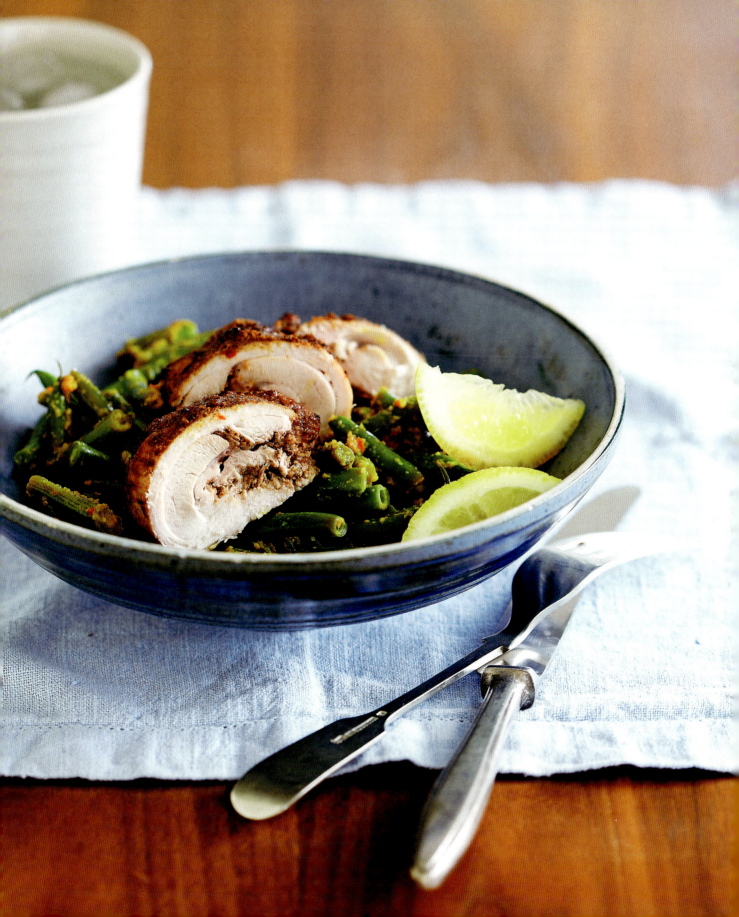

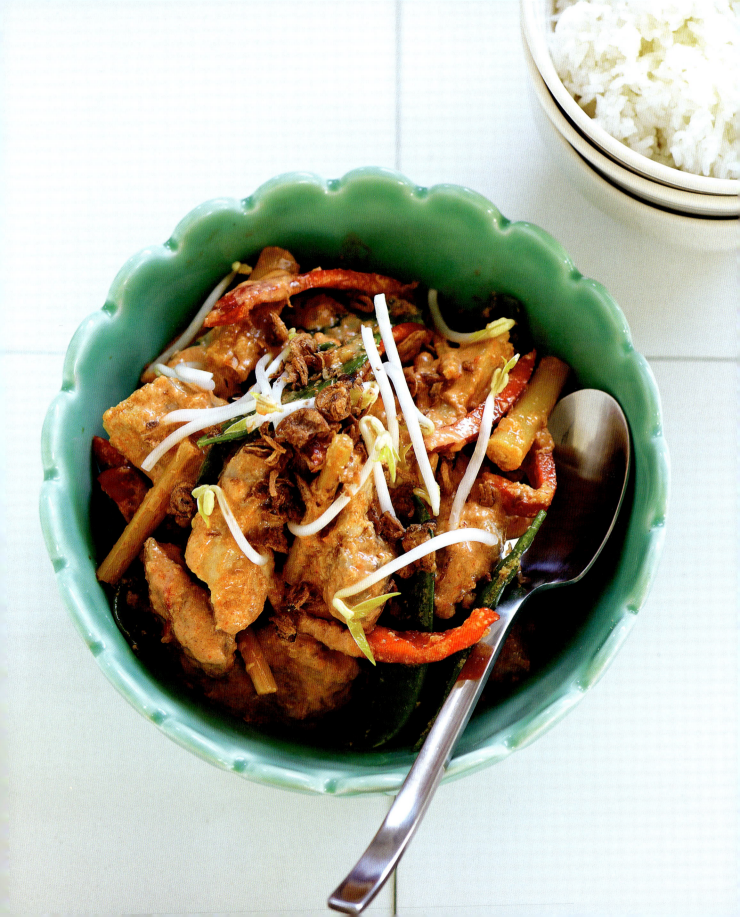

**2 units protein**
**¾ unit dairy**
**1½ units vegetables**
**1½ units fats**

2 teaspoons vegetable oil

4 red shallots or ½ red (Spanish) onion, finely chopped

3 cloves garlic, crushed

2 stalks lemongrass, bruised and chopped into 5 cm lengths

800 g skinless chicken thigh fillets, trimmed of fat and each piece cut into three

1–2 small red chillies, finely sliced

1½ tablespoons jungle curry or mild curry paste

1 teaspoon palm or brown sugar

1¼ cups (310 ml) reduced-fat coconut-flavoured evaporated milk

1½ tablespoons fish sauce

1 red capsicum (pepper), trimmed, seeded and thickly sliced

150 g snowpeas (mange-tout), trimmed

50 g bean sprouts, rinsed and drained

2 tablespoons fried shallots

# Chicken and lemongrass curry

SERVES 4  PREP **15 mins**  COOK **15 mins**

**Quick and simple to prepare, this curry is topped with fried shallots, a delicious crunchy garnish for curries and stir-fries that you can buy in packets from the supermarket.**

1  Place a large heavy-based saucepan over medium–high heat. Add the oil, shallot or onion, garlic and lemongrass and cook, stirring, for 2 minutes. Add the chicken, chilli, curry paste and sugar and cook for 4–5 minutes until the chicken is browned all over and well coated in the paste. Add the evaporated milk and fish sauce and stir to combine. Reduce the heat to low–medium, bring to simmering point and cook for 6–8 minutes until the chicken is cooked through.

2  Meanwhile, boil or steam the capsicum and snowpeas for 2 minutes until just tender, then drain and stir through the curry.

3  To serve, spoon the curry into bowls and garnish with the bean sprouts and fried shallots. Serve with steamed rice from your daily allowance if desired.

**Tip:** You can add any vegetables you have on hand to this curry – just cut them into similar sizes so they will all steam in the same amount of time. Alternatively, you could serve this with Braised Asian Vegetables on page 142 for 2 vegetable units.

# Indian-spiced roast chicken with warm carrot and radish salad

SERVES 4  PREP **15 mins, plus marinating time**  COOK **45 mins**

3 cloves garlic, finely chopped

2 tablespoons salt-reduced tomato paste (puree)

1½ tablespoons apple cider vinegar or white wine vinegar

1 tablespoon Garam Masala (see page 208)

1 tablespoon finely grated ginger

1 tablespoon coriander stems and roots, finely chopped

¼ teaspoon cayenne pepper

4 × 1.2 kg skinless chicken marylands (thigh and drumstick joints), trimmed of fat

lemon wedges and chopped coriander, to serve

**WARM CARROT AND RADISH SALAD**

3–4 carrots, grated

2 bunches radishes, trimmed, scrubbed and cut into 1 cm wedges

1 tablespoon vegetable oil

2 teaspoons mustard seeds

1 teaspoon cumin seeds

juice of ½ lemon

small handful coriander leaves, roughly chopped

**This beautifully spiced roast chicken needs to be marinated overnight for the flavours to fully develop. Roasting the chicken covered for the first 20 minutes of cooking time prevents the marinade from burning and the flesh from drying out before it's cooked all the way through. Use any leftover roast chicken in the Indian-spiced chicken wraps on page 139.**

1 Place the garlic, tomato paste, vinegar, garam masala, ginger, coriander stems and roots and cayenne pepper in a large shallow bowl and mix to combine. Add the chicken pieces, toss to coat and marinate in the fridge overnight.

2 Preheat the oven to 200°C.

3 Place the chicken on a baking-paper-lined baking tray, season with salt and pepper and cover with foil. Roast for 20 minutes, then remove the foil and roast for a further 20–25 minutes until cooked through.

4 Meanwhile, for the salad, bring a large saucepan of water to the boil and cook the carrot and radish for 5 minutes, then drain. Heat the vegetable oil in a large frying pan over high heat until almost smoking. Add the mustard and cumin seeds, then immediately remove the pan from the heat and stir for 30 seconds to prevent the spices from burning. Add the carrot and radish, then return to the heat and toss for 1 minute until coated in the seeds. Squeeze over the lemon juice, then season to taste with salt and pepper and scatter over the coriander.

5 Serve the chicken pieces with the salad, lemon wedges to the side and some chopped coriander scattered on top.

Tip: Use a hot curry powder instead of garam masala for a spicier result.

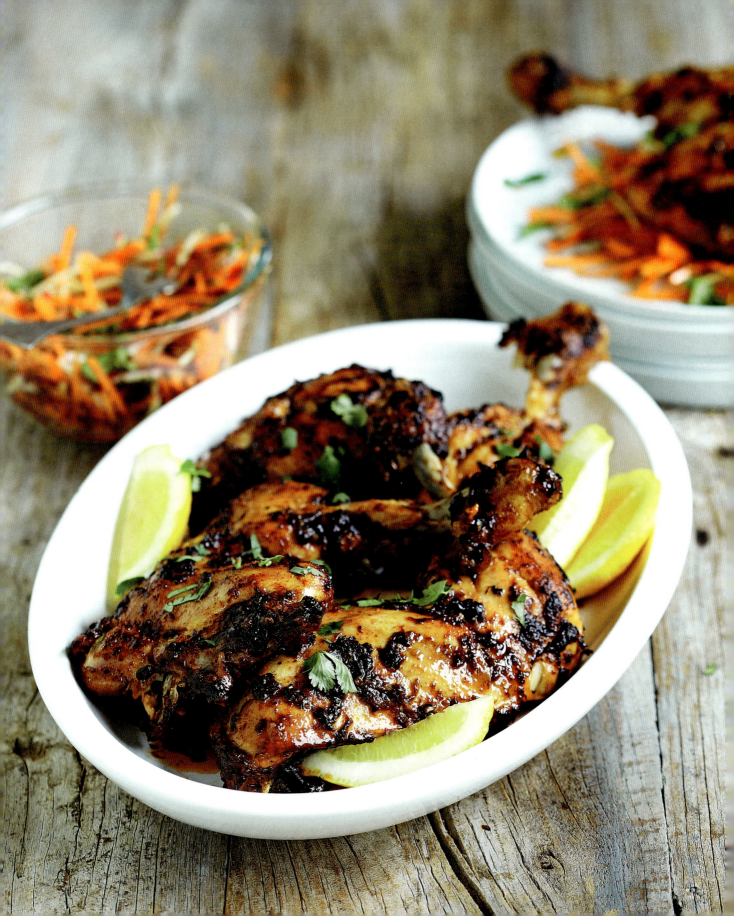

# Spice-rubbed chicken with tomato and green olive salad

SERVES 4  PREP **20 mins, plus marinating and standing time**
COOK **10 mins**

1½ tablespoons extra virgin olive oil
2 teaspoons smoked paprika
2 teaspoons ground cumin
1 teaspoon dried thyme
finely grated zest and juice of 1 lemon
800 g skinless chicken thigh fillets,
    trimmed of fat, cut into 3 cm pieces
300 g green beans, trimmed

**TOMATO AND GREEN OLIVE SALAD**
½ red (Spanish) onion, finely sliced
1 tablespoon extra virgin olive oil
1 small clove garlic, finely chopped
1 tablespoon red wine vinegar
½ teaspoon smoked paprika
600 g tomatoes, cut into 1 cm
    thick slices
60 g stuffed green olives, quartered

**Easy to prepare and cook, the chicken can be marinated overnight, making for a quick mid-week dinner.**

1 In a small bowl, combine 2 teaspoons of the olive oil with the smoked paprika, cumin, thyme, lemon zest and half the lemon juice and a few grinds of black pepper. Rub into the chicken and marinate for at least 30 minutes (or overnight if possible).

2 For the salad, soak the onion in a bowl of cold water for about 15 minutes, then drain. Combine the olive oil, garlic, vinegar and smoked paprika in a bowl and mix well. Add the tomato, olive and sliced onion, season to taste with salt and pepper combine gently. Leave to stand for 30 minutes at room temperature for the flavours to meld.

3 Heat a barbecue or chargrill pan to high. Season the chicken lightly with salt, then cook, turning, for 8–10 minutes until cooked through. Remove from the heat and pour over the remaining lemon juice.

4 Meanwhile, steam or boil the green beans for 3–4 minutes until just tender, then drain.

5 Serve the grilled chicken with the beans and plenty of tomato and green olive salad alongside.

# Red chicken curry with baby corn

SERVES 4  PREP **20 mins**  COOK **20 mins**

4 red shallots or ½ red (Spanish)
  onion, chopped
1 stalk lemongrass, white part only,
  finely chopped
1–2 small red chillies
1½ tablespoons ready-made
  Thai red curry paste
3 teaspoons ground coriander
1½ teaspoons ground cumin
1 tablespoon vegetable oil
800 g skinless chicken thigh fillets,
  trimmed of fat and cut into
  4 cm pieces
1 teaspoon palm or brown sugar
1¼ cups (310 ml) reduced-fat
  coconut-flavoured evaporated milk
1 tablespoon fish sauce
1 × 400 g tin baby corn, drained and
  halved lengthways
2 carrots, cut into very thin batons
½ lime, peeled and finely diced

**Adding some fresh ingredients to a ready-made curry paste adds depth and flavour to the finished dish.**

1 Blend the shallot or onion, lemongrass and chilli in a food processor until chopped. Add the curry paste, coriander and cumin, season with pepper and blend again until smooth.

2 Heat the oil in a heavy-based saucepan over medium heat. Fry the paste, stirring, for 6–7 minutes until it starts to darken and smells fragrant. Add the chicken and sugar and cook for 3–4 minutes until the chicken is browned all over. Stir in the evaporated milk and fish sauce, bring to simmering point and cook for 8 minutes. Add the corn and simmer for a further 2–3 minutes until the chicken is cooked through.

3 Meanwhile, steam or boil the carrots for 2 minutes until just tender, then drain and stir through the curry.

4 To serve, spoon the curry into bowls and scatter with diced lime. Serve with steamed rice from your daily allowance if desired.

2 units protein
¾ unit dairy
1½ units vegetables
1 unit fats

# Shellfish curry with tomato and lemongrass

SERVES 4  PREP **20 mins**  COOK **20 mins**

4 red shallots or ½ red (Spanish)
   onion, chopped
3 cloves garlic, chopped
1 stalk lemongrass, white part
   chopped, green part bruised
1½ tablespoons ready-made
   Thai yellow curry paste
3 tomatoes, chopped
1 teaspoon ground coriander
1 teaspoon ground turmeric
1¼ cups (310 ml) reduced-fat
   coconut-flavoured evaporated milk
1½ tablespoons fish sauce
400 g green beans, trimmed
200 g white fish fillets (such as blue-
   eye, ling or snapper), skin and
   bones removed, cut into 5 cm pieces
1 kg mussels, scrubbed
   and debearded
2 tablespoons chopped coriander

**The addition of tomato to this Vietnamese-style curry adds a gentle sweetness which works equally well with any white-fleshed fish, shellfish or chicken. If the curry is a little thick, add an extra 3 tablespoons evaporated milk (this will add ¼ unit dairy).**

1 Blend the shallot or onion, garlic and chopped lemongrass in a food processor until finely chopped. Add the curry paste and a small handful of the chopped tomato and blend to a smooth paste. Add the remaining tomato and blend until smooth. Stir in the ground spices and season with black pepper.

2 Place a large heavy-based saucepan over medium–high heat and add the curry paste. Bring to the boil, stirring, then reduce the heat to low–medium and cook for 8–10 minutes, stirring regularly, until aromatic. Add the evaporated milk, fish sauce and the bruised lemongrass, bring to simmering point and cook for 5 minutes (do not let the mixture boil). Add the green beans and cook for 2 minutes, then add the fish and cook for a further 4–5 minutes until the beans are tender and the fish is cooked through.

3 Meanwhile, bring 1 cup (250 ml) water to the boil in a large saucepan or stockpot, then add the mussels, cover and cook for 5 minutes until the mussels open.

4 To serve, divide the fish and green beans among four bowls, top with the mussels and ladle over the sauce. Scatter with coriander, and serve with rice from your daily allowance if desired.

**Tip:** For a spicier curry, add 2–3 chopped bird's-eye chillies when blending the paste.

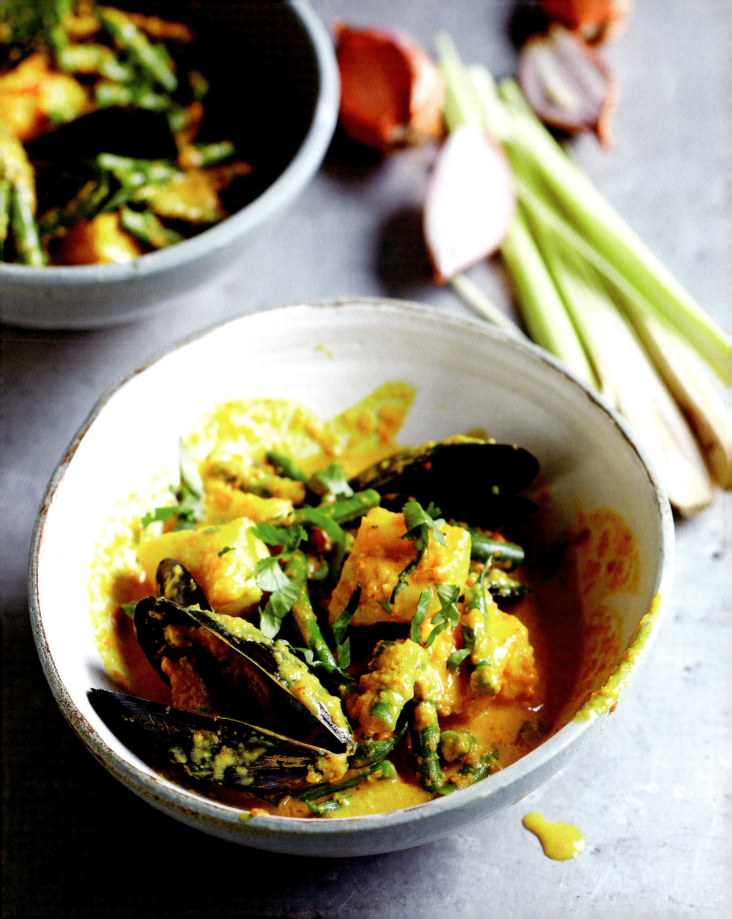

**1 SERVE =**

2 units protein

2 units vegetables

2 units fats

# Slow-baked chicken with black olives, tomato and oregano

SERVES 4  PREP **15 mins**  COOK **1 hour 40 mins**

cooking oil spray

800 g skinless chicken thigh fillets,
   trimmed of fat and halved

1 tablespoon olive oil

1 onion, finely chopped

2 carrots, chopped

2 sticks celery, chopped

1 tablespoon dried oregano
   or Italian herbs

250 g button mushrooms, quartered

2 cloves garlic, finely chopped

1 × 400 g tin peeled tomatoes

$^2/_3$ cup (80 g) black olives

2 tablespoons salt-reduced tomato
   paste (puree)

small handful basil leaves (optional)

Pumpkin and Sweet Potato Mash
   (see page 149), to serve

**Rich, thick and intensely flavoured, this Italian classic is sure to please.**

1 Preheat the oven to 170°C.

2 Heat a large heavy-based saucepan over medium–high heat and spray with cooking oil. Working in batches, cook the chicken for 2–3 minutes until browned on all sides. Remove from the pan and set aside.

3 Reduce the heat to medium and add the olive oil. When hot, add the onion, carrot, celery and dried herbs and cook, stirring occasionally, for 8–10 minutes until the vegetables are soft. Add the mushrooms and garlic and cook for 2 minutes. Add the tomatoes, olives and tomato paste, then season to taste with salt and pepper and stir to combine. Return the chicken to the pan. Bring to the boil, then cover and transfer to the oven for 1 hour. Remove the lid and cook for a further 15–20 minutes until the chicken is tender and the sauce has reduced. Scatter over the basil, if using, and serve with mash.

Tip: You can also cook this on the stovetop – just keep the heat as low as possible (use a simmer mat if you have one) so the chicken cooks very gently (the exact cooking time will vary depending on the heat setting: check after 1 hour and continue until the chicken is cooked through and tender).

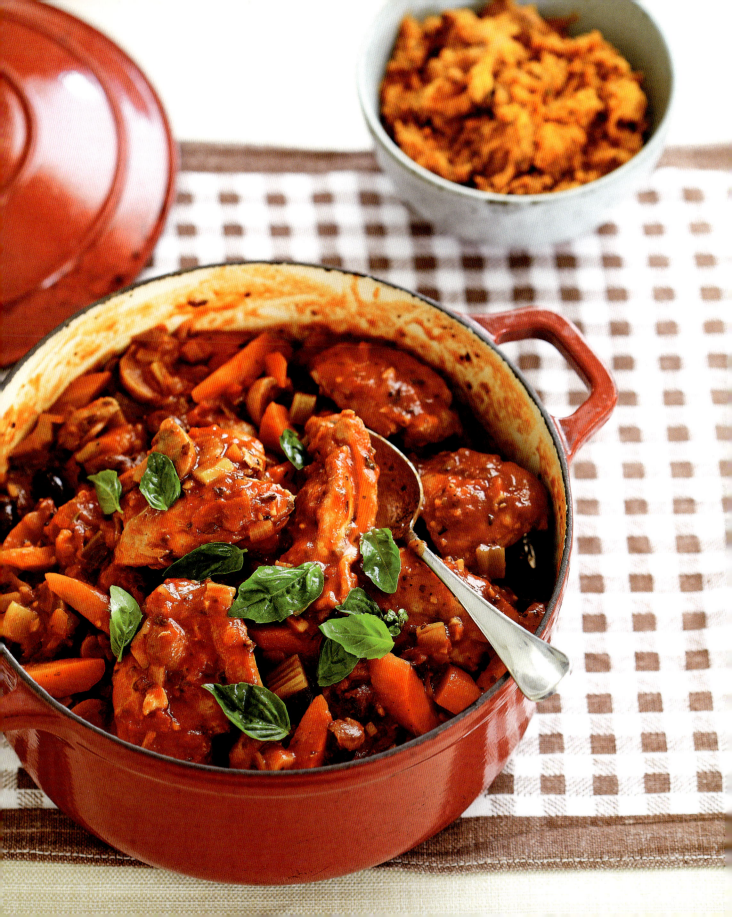

1 SERVE =
**2 units protein**
**1½ units bread**
**1½ units vegetables**
**1½ units fats**

1 kg plain flour
1 × 1.5 kg chicken, skin removed
   with a sharp knife
1 lemon, halved
2 tablespoons finely chopped
   flat-leaf parsley
2 teaspoons extra virgin olive oil
1 tablespoon thyme leaves or
   2 teaspoons dried thyme
4 cloves garlic, 3 crushed, 1 whole

**LENTIL SALAD**
1 carrot, cut into 5 mm dice
150 g green beans, sliced into
   5 mm rounds
1 zucchini (courgette), cut into
   5 mm dice
1 tablespoon olive oil
2 cloves garlic, finely chopped
1 long red chilli, seeded and
   finely sliced
1½ cups (280 g) cooked
   lentils, warmed
1 tablespoon Dijon mustard
1 tablespoon red wine vinegar

# Chicken baked in a bread crust with lentil salad

SERVES 4  PREP **30 mins**  COOK **90 mins, plus resting time**

**Enclosing the chicken in a bread crust seals in the moisture and prevents any flavour escaping during cooking. The result is succulent, juicy and fragrant chicken, with enough leftovers for the best sandwiches ever (see page 137).**

1 Preheat the oven to 200°C and line a baking tray with baking paper.

2 Combine the flour and 1½ cups (375 ml) warm water in a bowl and mix until the dough starts to come together. Gradually add an extra ½ cup (125 ml) warm water, mixing between additions, until the dough is pliable but not too sticky, then set aside.

3 Zest and juice one of the lemon halves and slice the other half. In a small bowl, combine the lemon juice, zest, parsley, olive oil, thyme and ¾ of the crushed garlic. Season with salt and pepper and rub this marinade all over the chicken. Place the lemon slices and the remaining clove of garlic inside the cavity of the chicken.

4 Divide the dough in half and roll each portion into a 33 cm diameter circle. Sit the chicken in the centre of one dough round and drape the other round over the top. Bring the edges of each round together and pinch to seal.

5 Place the chicken on the prepared tray and bake for 1½ hours. Remove from the oven and set aside to rest for 15 minutes.

6 For the lentil salad, steam or boil the vegetables together in a large saucepan for 2 minutes until just tender, then drain. Place a saucepan over medium heat, add the olive oil, garlic and chilli and cook for 2–3 minutes until the garlic softens. Add the lentils, mustard, vinegar and vegetables and cook, stirring, for 1 minute until combined and heated through.

7 Gently crack the bread crust, being careful to save some of the juices trapped inside. Remove the chicken and discard the crust. Carve the chicken and serve 200 g per person, with the juices drizzled over and the lentil salad to the side.

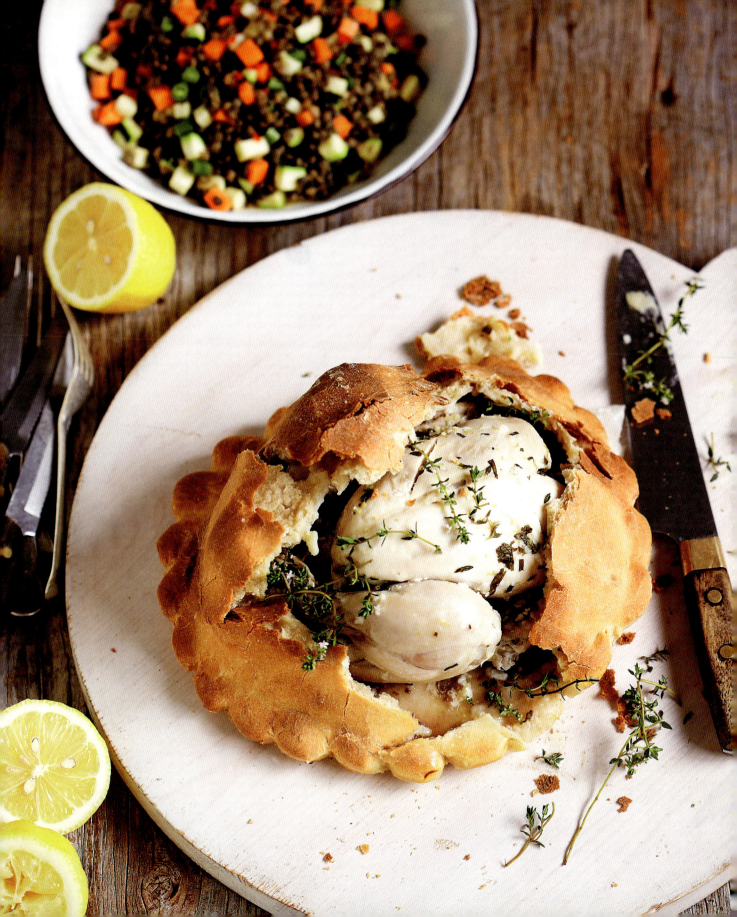

# SLOW-COOKER RECIPES

# Lamb shanks with braised carrots and roast parsnips

SERVES 4  PREP **15 mins**  COOK **8 hours**

4 lamb shanks, trimmed of fat
cooking oil spray
1 tablespoon olive oil
1 onion, roughly chopped
3 cloves garlic, chopped
2 sprigs rosemary, leaves stripped
    or 3 teaspoons dried rosemary
2 tablespoons salt-reduced tomato
    paste (puree)
2 cups (500 ml) Chicken Stock
    (see page 209)
1 carrot, cut into 3 cm pieces
2 teaspoons smoked paprika,
    plus extra to sprinkle
400 g parsnips, peeled, trimmed and
    halved lengthways
2 teaspoons honey, warmed
Garlic and Mint Pea Puree (see page
    148), to serve

**A much-loved classic, this recipe is rich and loaded with flavour. Make sure you skim off the fat from the surface of the braise after cooking. Add a couple of extra shanks and use the leftovers in the lamb burekas on page 124.**

1 Place a large frying pan over high heat. Spray the shanks with cooking oil and fry in two batches for 7–8 minutes or until browned on all sides, then transfer to the slow-cooker.

2 Reduce the heat to medium, then add the olive oil, onion, garlic and rosemary and cook, stirring occasionally, for 4–5 minutes until the onion starts to soften. Add the tomato paste and cook, stirring, for 1 minute. Add ½ cup (125 ml) of the chicken stock and stir to combine, scraping the bottom of the pan, then tip this mixture into the slow-cooker. Add the remaining stock, the carrots and paprika, season with salt and pepper and stir to combine. Cover and cook on low for 7–8 hours or until the lamb is almost falling off the bone. Skim away any fat from the surface.

3 About an hour before you're ready to eat, preheat the oven to 220°C and line a baking tray with baking paper. Arrange the parsnips on the prepared tray and spray with cooking oil. Drizzle over the honey, season with black pepper and sprinkle with a pinch of extra paprika. Roast for 50–60 minutes until the parsnips are golden and crisp.

4 Serve the shanks with the carrots and warmed pea puree, and spoon over some sauce. Serve with roast parsnips alongside.

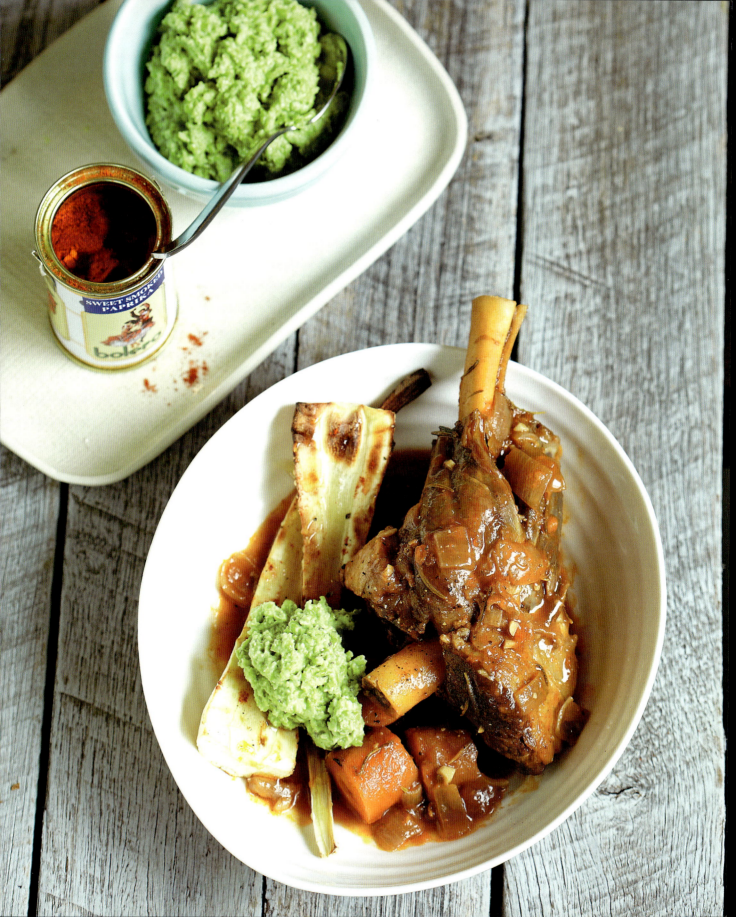

# Fragrant chicken with pickled radish salad

SERVES 4   PREP **15 mins, plus marinating time**   COOK **5 hours**

**Taking its cues from the flavours of the Caribbean, this aromatic chicken dish is succulent and juicy. Refrigerate overnight before cooking so the marinade has time to penetrate the chicken.**

1 brown onion, roughly chopped
4 cloves garlic, roughly chopped
3–4 small red chillies,
   roughly chopped
1 tablespoon salt-reduced tomato
   paste (puree)
1 tablespoon brown vinegar
   or malt vinegar
1 tablespoons thyme leaves or
   2 teaspoons dried thyme
1½ teaspoons ground allspice
¾ teaspoon ground cinnamon
1 kg skinless chicken drumsticks
3–4 sticks celery, cut into
   5 cm lengths
1½ cups (375 ml) Chicken Stock
   (see page 209)

**PICKLED RADISH SALAD**
200 g sugar snap peas
200 g iceberg lettuce (about ½ head),
   washed and torn
75 g Pickled Radish (see page 201)
   or ½ bunch radishes, trimmed
   and thinly sliced
1 × 250 g punnet cherry
   tomatoes, halved
1 quantity Paprika and Honey
   Dressing (see page 206)

1 In a food processor, combine the onion, garlic, chilli and tomato paste and process until finely chopped. Add the vinegar and process until smooth. Mix in the herbs and spices, season with black pepper and combine well. Place the chicken pieces in a large, shallow dish and cover with the marinade. Cover and refrigerate overnight.

2 Arrange the celery over the base of the slow-cooker and place the chicken and any remaining marinade on top. Season with salt, pour in the stock, then cover and cook on low for 4–5 hours until the chicken is tender.

3 Meanwhile, for the salad, blanch the sugar snaps in a saucepan of boiling water for 2 minutes until bright green and tender. Drain, refresh in cold water, then drain again. Place in a large bowl with the lettuce, radish and cherry tomatoes, pour over the dressing and toss to combine.

4 To serve, spoon the celery onto plates and top with chicken pieces and sauce. Serve with the pickled radish salad.

800 g skinless chicken thighs, trimmed of fat
2 teaspoons sweet paprika
cooking oil spray
1 tablespoon olive oil
1 large leek, trimmed, washed and cut into 1 cm thick rounds
1 teaspoon fennel seeds
2 teaspoons dried sage
3 cloves garlic, crushed
300 g potato, cut into 3 cm pieces
finely grated zest of 1 lemon
1½ cups (375 ml) Chicken Stock (see page 209)

**SQUASH AND FETA SALAD**
cooking oil spray
6 yellow patty pan squash (about 240 g), cut into 1 cm thick slices
2 zucchinis (courgettes), cut into 1 cm thick rounds
80 g feta
2 teaspoons drained capers
juice of 1 lemon

# Garlic and sage chicken with squash and feta salad

SERVES 4  PREP **15 mins**  COOK **4½ hours**

**Garlic and sage are perfect partners to the humble chicken. Plan ahead and make a double batch of this to use in the chicken pie recipe on page 130.**

1 Dust the chicken with 1 teaspoon of the paprika. Spray a large frying pan with cooking oil and heat over medium–high heat. Working in batches if necessary, cook the chicken thighs for 3–4 minutes until browned all over. Remove and set aside.

2 Reduce the heat to medium and add the olive oil, leek, fennel seeds and sage. Cook for 5–6 minutes until the leek begins to soften. Add the garlic and cook for 2 minutes, then transfer this mixture to the slow-cooker, along with the potato, lemon zest, chicken stock and the remaining paprika. Season to taste with salt and pepper and stir to combine. Place the browned chicken pieces on top, then cover and cook on low for 4–4½ hours until the chicken is tender and the potato is cooked.

3 Meanwhile, for the salad, spray a chargrill pan with cooking oil and heat over medium–high heat. Cook the squash and zucchini for 5–6 minutes, turning regularly, until tender. Place in a large bowl, along with the feta, capers and lemon juice. Season to taste with salt and pepper and toss to combine.

4 To serve, divide the leek and potato among four plates and top with the chicken. Spoon over some sauce and serve with the squash and feta salad.

# Pork braised with beans, tomato and chilli

SERVES 4 PREP **10 mins, plus soaking time** COOK **7 hours**

1 cup (195 g) dried white beans
cooking oil spray
1 × 800 g pork shoulder, trimmed
    of fat and cut into 3 cm pieces
1 tablespoon olive oil
1 onion, chopped
3 cloves garlic, finely chopped
2–3 long red chillies, finely sliced
2 bay leaves
2 sprigs rosemary or
    1–2 tablespoons dried rosemary
1 cup (250 ml) Chicken Stock
    (see page 209) or water
375 g salt-reduced tomato passata
    (preferably with fresh herbs added)
2 bunches broccolini,
    cut into large florets
finely grated zest and juice of 1 lemon

**Browning the pork and cooking the aromatics first helps to build a great flavour base for the braise, but if time is tight, simply combine everything in the slow-cooker and turn the switch to low. The white beans will need to be soaked overnight before cooking.**

1 Soak the beans in water overnight, then drain.

2 Spray a large frying pan with cooking oil and place over high heat. Working in batches, cook the pork for 3–4 minutes until browned on all sides, then transfer to the slow-cooker.

3 Reduce the heat to medium and add the olive oil, onion, garlic, chilli and bay leaves. Cook, stirring, for 5 minutes until the onion begins to soften, then add this mixture to the slow-cooker, along with the beans, rosemary, chicken stock and passata. Season with pepper and stir to combine, then cover and cook on low for 6–7 hours or until the pork and beans are tender.

4 Steam or boil the broccolini until just tender. Toss with the lemon juice and grind over some pepper.

5 To serve, spoon the pork and beans into bowls, then top with lemon zest and serve with broccolini alongside.

**Tip:** Garnish with some chopped flat-leaf parsley if you have it to hand. You can use broccoli if you can't get broccolini.

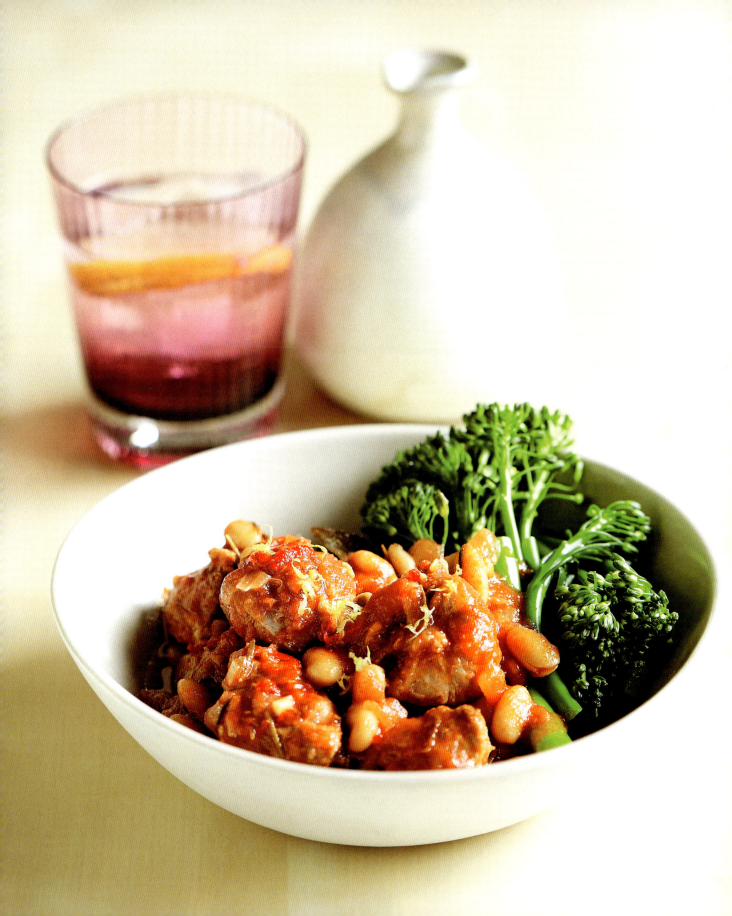

cooking oil spray
800 g chuck steak, trimmed of fat
    and cut into 3 cm pieces
1 tablespoon olive oil
12 whole pickling onions, peeled
    or 2 small onions, chopped
300 g carrots, chopped into
    2 cm pieces
300 g potato, chopped into 3 cm pieces
3 cloves garlic, chopped
1–2 tablespoons dried Italian herbs
2 cups (500 ml) salt-reduced
    beef stock
1 tablespoon Vegemite
1½ tablespoons Worcestershire sauce
1 tablespoon salt-reduced tomato
    paste (puree)
Parsnip and Cauliflower Puree
    (see page 149), to serve

# Rich beef stew

SERVES 4  PREP **20 mins**  COOK **7 hours**

**A warming winter favourite. Make a double batch and turn this hearty stew into a filo-topped pie following the recipe on page 126.**

1 Spray a large frying pan with cooking oil and place over medium–high heat. Working in batches, cook the beef until browned on all sides, then transfer to the slow-cooker.

2 Reduce the heat to medium, add the olive oil, onion, carrot and potato and cook for 7–8 minutes until the vegetables begin to soften. Add the garlic and herbs and cook for another 2 minutes, then transfer this mixture to the slow-cooker. Add ½ cup (125 ml) of the stock to the frying pan, along with the Vegemite, and stir over medium heat to dissolve, then add this to the slow-cooker, along with the Worcestershire sauce, tomato paste and remaining stock. Season with pepper and stir to combine. Cover and cook on low for 6–7 hours until the beef and vegetables are tender.

3 Divide the warm cauliflower and parsnip puree among plates or bowls and top with the beef and vegetables. Spoon over some sauce and serve.

**Tip:** Try replacing the stock with a 375 ml can of stout or Guinness for a different flavour.

# Oregano and lemon chicken with Greek salad

SERVES 4  PREP **20 mins**  COOK **4 hours 30 mins**

cooking oil spray
800 g skinless chicken thighs,
    trimmed of fat
2 teaspoons olive oil
1 red (Spanish) onion, finely sliced
3 cloves garlic, finely chopped
2 sprigs thyme or 1 teaspoon
    dried thyme
2 teaspoons dried oregano
finely grated zest and juice of 1 lemon
1 cup (250 ml) Chicken Stock
    (see page 209)
4 tablespoons risoni
40 g reduced-fat feta

**GREEK SALAD**
juice of 1 lemon
1 tablespoon extra virgin olive oil
1 cos lettuce, washed, leaves torn
4 roma (plum) tomatoes,
    cut into wedges
1 Lebanese (small) cucumber,
    cut into 1 cm pieces
10 medium-sized black olives, halved
120 g reduced-fat feta, cut into
    1 cm cubes

**Cooking the risoni with the chicken means it soaks up all the delicious cooking juices. Add a few extra chicken thighs to the slow-cooker to use in the caesar salad recipe on page 127.**

1  Spray a large frying pan with cooking oil and heat over medium–high heat. Working in batches, brown the chicken pieces on all sides for 3–4 minutes, then transfer to the slow-cooker.

2  Reduce the heat to medium and add the olive oil, onion, garlic, thyme and oregano. Cook, stirring occasionally, for 7–8 minutes until the onion is soft but not coloured. Add this mixture to the slow-cooker along with the lemon juice and chicken stock. Season to taste with salt and pepper and stir to combine. Cover and cook on low for 4 hours or until the chicken is very tender. Remove the lid, quickly stir through the risoni, ensuring it is submerged in the stock, then cover and cook for a further 15 minutes.

3  Meanwhile, for the salad, combine the lemon juice and olive oil and season with pepper. Combine the rest of the ingredients in a bowl and toss through the dressing.

4  To serve, divide the chicken and risoni among plates or bowls. Crumble over the feta and sprinkle with the reserved lemon zest. Serve with the Greek salad.

**Tip:** If you have fresh oregano on hand, stir 2 chopped tablespoons through the chicken before serving.

# USING
## LEFTOVERS

2 bulbs fennel, trimmed, fronds
   roughly chopped and reserved,
   bulbs cut into 5 mm slices
cooking oil spray
400 g shredded braised lamb shanks
   (from Lamb Shanks with Braised
   Carrots and Roast Parsnips on
   page 114)
225 g frozen spinach
2 teaspoons fennel seeds
2 tablespoons raisins, chopped
160 g reduced-fat feta
2 teaspoons ground cinnamon
4 sheets filo pastry
2 oranges, peeled and
   white pith removed
120 g rocket leaves
1 tablespoon extra virgin olive oil
3 teaspoons white wine vinegar

**Tip:** If the weather's cold, serve these
burekas with ½ portion Carrot Puree
(see page 148) for ½ vegetable unit.

# Lamb burekas with fennel and orange salad

SERVES 4  PREP **20 mins**  COOK **50 mins**

**Rich, crisp, and flaky, burekas are the Middle Eastern version of a sausage roll (without the tomato sauce, of course), and make for a delicious lunch. Use leftovers from the braised lamb shank recipe.**

1 Preheat the oven to 200°C and line one or two baking trays with baking paper.

2 Place the sliced fennel in a single layer on the prepared tray/s, season to taste with salt and pepper and spray with cooking oil. Roast for 20–25 minutes until tender and golden. Remove from the oven and, when cool enough to handle, roughly chop ¼ of the fennel, reserving the rest for the salad. Reduce the oven temperature to 180°C.

3 In a large bowl, combine the chopped roast fennel and fronds, the shredded lamb, spinach, fennel seeds, raisins, feta and cinnamon. Season to taste with salt and pepper and mix well.

4 Spray a sheet of filo pastry with cooking oil and fold in half lengthways. Spoon ¼ of the lamb mixture along one long edge, leaving a 5 cm border. Fold in the short edges, then fold to enclose. Spray again with cooking oil. Repeat with the remaining filo sheets and lamb.

5 Place the burekas on the prepared trays, seam-side down, and cook for 20–25 minutes until lightly golden and crisp.

6 Meanwhile, segment the oranges by holding them over a bowl and, using a small, sharp knife, cut the flesh away from the inner membrane, letting the segments and any juice fall into the bowl. Place the segments in another bowl with the reserved roast fennel and rocket. Mix together the olive oil, vinegar and 2 tablespoons of the orange juice, season to taste, then add to the salad and toss to combine.

7 Serve the burekas with some salad.

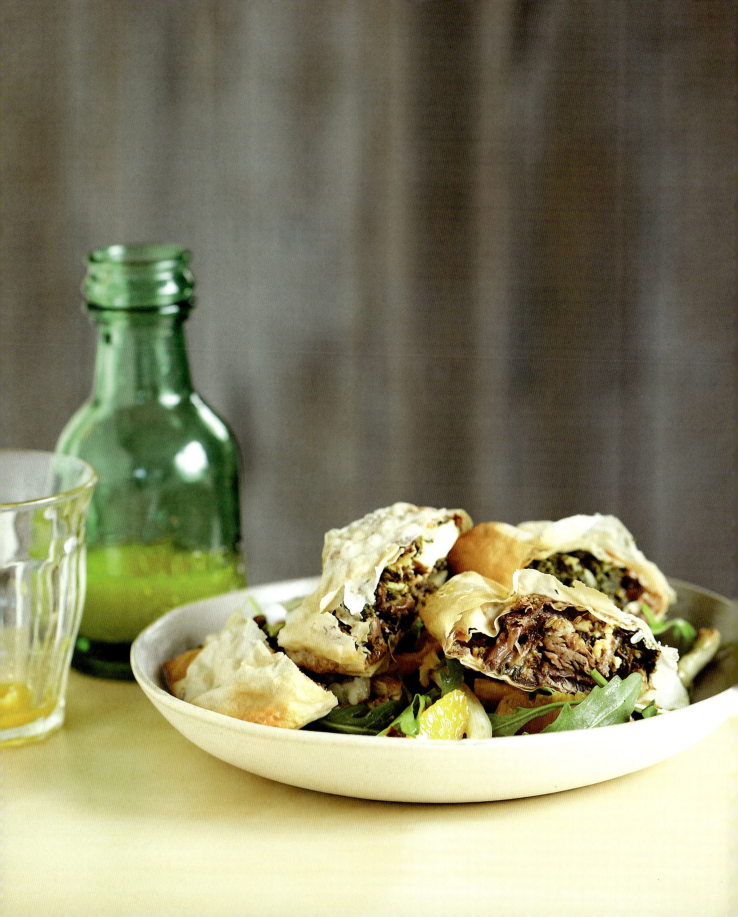

1 quantity Rich Beef Stew
   (see page 120)
1 tablespoon plain flour
cooking oil spray
4 sheets filo pastry
Sumac-spiced Broccoli and Peas
   (see page 152) and Tomato and
   Onion Salad (see page 155), to serve

# Beef pie

SERVES 4  PREP **15 mins**  COOK **30 mins**

**Everybody loves a good pie, but we don't always have the time to make them. This delicious pie features leftover stew as the filling, making it not only economical but a cinch to prepare on a busy weeknight.**

1 Preheat the oven to 180°C.

2 In a large saucepan, reheat the beef stew over low–medium heat. Using a slotted spoon, transfer the beef to a plate and chop into small chunks. Bring the remaining sauce and vegetables to simmering point, then roughly crush the vegetables with a potato masher. Mix the flour with 1 tablespoon water to make a smooth paste, then stir this into the sauce. Cook over low heat for 1–2 minutes until the mixture thickens. Return the beef to the pan, stir to combine and season with salt and pepper.

3 Spray a 1.5 litre ovenproof dish with cooking oil, then spoon the beef mixture into the dish. Lay the filo sheets out on a clean work surface and spray with cooking oil. Arrange the filo sheets on top of the beef, place the dish in the oven and bake for 20–25 minutes until the pastry is golden and crisp.

4 Serve the pie with the vegetables and salad to the side.

**Tip:** For an added lift, try stirring some chopped roast vegetables like fennel, cauliflower or onion into the filling before baking.

**2 units protein**
**1 unit bread**
**1 unit dairy**
**1 unit vegetables**
**1 unit fats**

2 slices sourdough bread,
cut into 1 cm cubes
cooking oil spray
150 g lean rindless bacon,
sliced into thin batons
4 anchovy fillets, drained of oil
and finely chopped
1 small clove garlic, chopped
1 quantity Salad Cream
(see page 207)
400 g Oregano and Lemon Chicken
(see page 121), meat removed
from the bones and shredded into
large pieces
1 cos lettuce, leaves separated
and torn
1 × 250 g punnet cherry
tomatoes, halved
80 g parmesan, shaved
4 soft-boiled eggs

# Oregano and lemon chicken caesar salad

SERVES 4  PREP **10 mins**  COOK **8 mins**

**This classic salad features the lemony braised chicken thighs from page 121 (or you could use any cooked chicken). The chicken should be at room temperature to make the most of the flavours.**

1 Preheat the oven to 200°C and line a baking tray with baking paper.

2 Place the cubes of bread on the prepared tray and spray with cooking oil. Bake for 8–10 minutes until crisp, then set aside.

3 Heat a medium-sized frying pan over medium–high heat and spray with cooking oil. Add the bacon and cook, stirring now and then, for 5–6 minutes until crisp, then drain on paper towel and set aside.

4 Using a mortar and pestle, pound the anchovies and garlic to a smooth paste. Prepare the salad cream dressing and add this paste and some pepper, mixing well to combine.

5 Place the chicken, lettuce, tomato, half the cheese and half the croutons in a large bowl, pour over the dressing and toss well to combine. Divide the salad among four plates and top each with a soft-boiled egg, some bacon and the remaining cheese and croutons.

Tip: Leave the anchovies out if you don't like them – the salad will still be delicious.

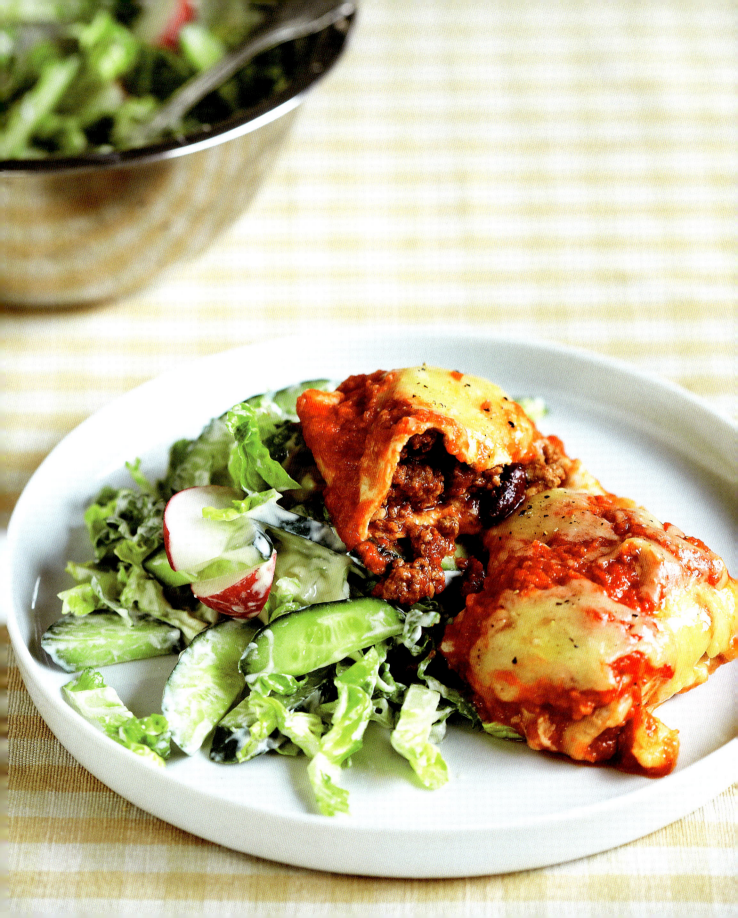

# Enchiladas with radish and cucumber salad

SERVES 4 PREP **20 mins** COOK **40 mins**

1 quantity Garlic Yoghurt Dressing
  (see page 207)
½ teaspoon dried mint
2 teaspoons olive oil
½ onion, chopped
2 cloves garlic, chopped
½ teaspoon ground cumin
¼ teaspoon ground allspice
1 × 400 g tin chopped tomatoes
cooking oil spray
4 wholemeal tortillas
½ quantity cooled Chilli Con Carne
  (see page 63)
160 g reduced-fat tasty cheese, grated
6–8 drops Tabasco sauce
1 bunch radishes, trimmed, scrubbed
  and sliced into thin wedges
2 Lebanese (small) cucumbers,
  quartered lengthways, sliced
½–1 cos lettuce (225 g), shredded

**You can make these spicy little numbers for lunch using leftover chilli con carne. Prepare the tomato sauce in advance, then when you're almost ready to eat, just assemble the enchiladas and pop them in the oven. If time is tight, use a ready-made tomato passata with the spices stirred through.**

1 Preheat the oven to 200°C.

2 Prepare the dressing, then stir in the mint. Set aside for the flavours to infuse.

3 Place a small saucepan over medium heat. Add the olive oil, onion and garlic and cook for 4–5 minutes until the onion softens. Add the ground spices and cook for 1 minute, then add the tomato and season with salt and pepper to taste. Reduce the heat to low–medium and simmer for 10 minutes until thickened. Transfer to a blender and blend until smooth.

4 Spray a 1.5 litre, 22 cm square ovenproof dish with cooking oil and spoon in ¼ of the tomato sauce. Lay out the tortillas on a clean work surface. Divide the chilli con carne among the tortillas and sprinkle with ¼ of the cheese, reserving the rest. Roll up each enchilada and place seam-side down in the dish. Spoon over the remaining tomato sauce, sprinkle over the remaining cheese and dot with Tabasco. Place in the oven and cook for 20–25 minutes until the cheese is melted and bubbling.

5 Combine the radish, cucumber and cos lettuce in a bowl, pour over the dressing and toss to combine.

6 Serve the enchiladas with salad alongside.

# Garlic and sage chicken pie

SERVES 4  PREP **15 mins**  COOK **30 mins**

1 quantity Garlic and Sage Chicken
(see page 117)

1 carrot, chopped into 5 mm pieces

1 cup (120 g) frozen peas

finely grated zest and juice of 1 lemon

4 sheets filo pastry

cooking oil spray

**Braised Green Beans with Tomato and
Oregano (see page 146), to serve**

**Another quick and easy pie, this one uses garlic and sage
chicken as its filling. The addition of fresh peas and lemon
gives it a lift.**

1 Preheat the oven to 180°C.

2 Reheat the chicken mixture in a covered saucepan over low–
medium heat. Using a slotted spoon, transfer the chicken to
a plate, remove the meat from the bone and chop the meat into
small chunks. Mash the potato in the saucepan to a chunky
mash, then return the chicken to the pan.

3 Steam or boil the carrots for 3–4 minutes until tender, then drain
and add to the chicken mixture, along with the peas, lemon zest
and 2 tablespoons of the lemon juice. Season to taste with salt
and pepper and mix gently to combine, being careful not to break
up the chicken.

4 Spray a 1.5 litre ovenproof dish with cooking oil, then spoon the
chicken mixture into the dish. Lay out the filo sheets on a clean
work surface and spray with cooking oil. Arrange the filo sheets
on top of the chicken, then place the dish in the oven and bake
for 20–25 minutes until the pastry is golden and crisp.

5 Serve the pie with braised beans.

**Tip:** Add 2 tablespoons chopped fresh herbs such as flat-leaf parsley,
chives or sage to the chicken mixture before baking.

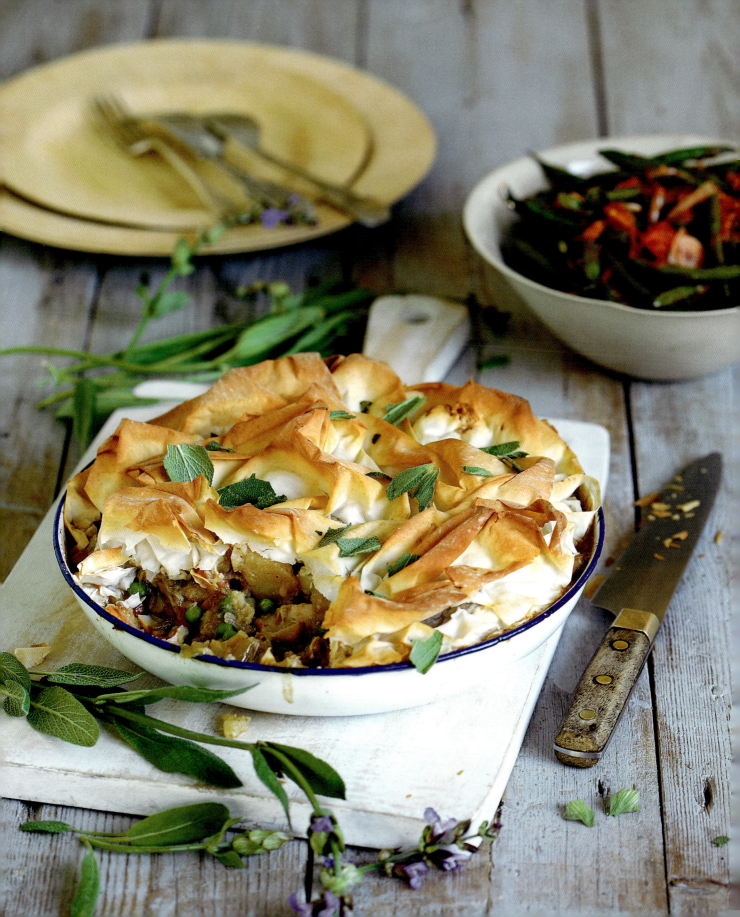

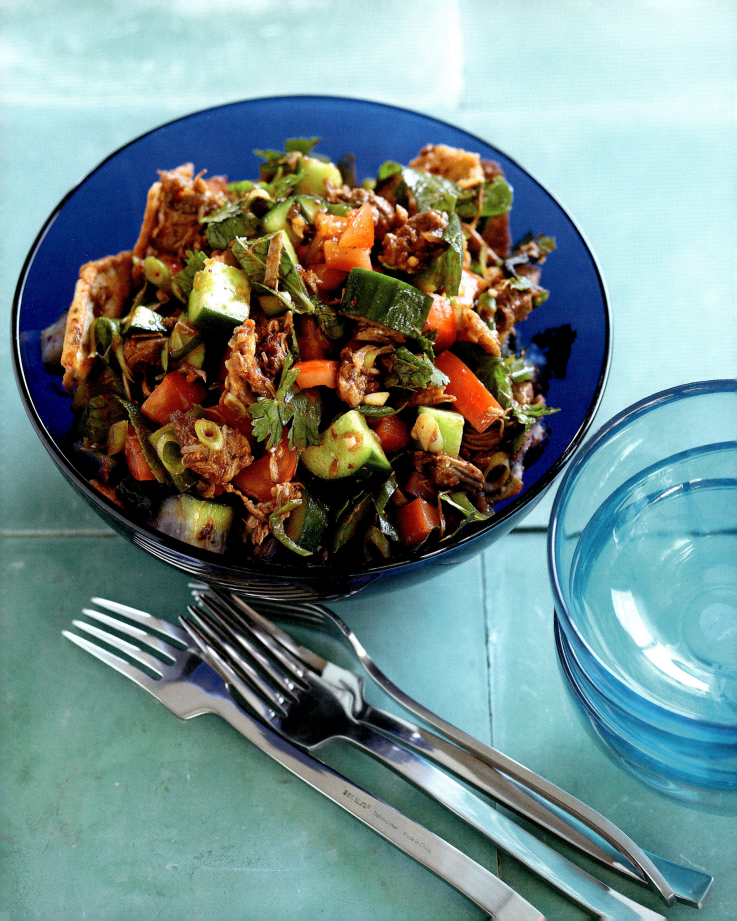

**1 SERVE =**
1 unit protein
½ unit bread
2 units vegetables
1 unit fats

2 small wholemeal pita breads
cooking oil spray
½ teaspoon ground sumac
400 g Braised Lamb Shoulder
    (see page 84), shredded
4 small tomatoes, diced
1 green capsicum (pepper), diced
2 Lebanese (small) cucumbers, diced
4 spring onions, trimmed and sliced
handful chopped mixed herbs, such
    as mint, coriander and parsley

**SUMAC DRESSING**
1 tablespoon extra virgin olive oil
2 tablespoons lemon juice
1 small clove garlic, crushed
½ teaspoon ground sumac

# Fattoush salad with lamb

SERVES 4  PREP **15 mins**  COOK **15 mins**

**Fattoush is a Middle Eastern salad made with toasted pita bread and spiced with sumac. The addition of lamb makes it a hearty lunch. This recipe uses leftovers from the braised lamb shoulder recipe (or you could use any cooked lamb). Don't add the pita crisps to the salad until the last minute so they stay nice and crunchy.**

1 Preheat the oven to 180°C and line a baking tray with baking paper.

2 For the dressing, combine all the ingredients in a jar, season to taste with salt and pepper and shake well. Set aside to allow the flavours to infuse.

3 Place the pitas on the prepared tray, spray them with cooking oil and sprinkle over the sumac. Bake for 5–6 minutes until crisp, then remove from the oven and reduce the oven temperature to 150°C. When the pitas are cool enough to handle, break them into small shards and set aside.

4 Add the lamb to the tray, cover with foil and place in the oven for 10 minutes, just so the lamb is warm enough to loosen a little.

5 Place the tomato, capsicum, cucumber, spring onion and lamb in a large bowl. Add the dressing and chopped herbs and toss to combine. Just before serving, gently stir through the pita crisps.

**Tip:** Add 80 g feta for 1 dairy unit.

# Spring rolls with Asian slaw

**SERVES** 4  PREP **20 mins**  COOK **25 mins**

These spring rolls, using leftovers from the san choi bao recipe, are baked rather than fried. Enjoy them for a flavour-packed lunch.

4 sheets filo pastry
cooking oil spray
½ quantity pork filling from Thai-style San Choi Bao (see page 92)
2 cups (150 g) finely shredded white cabbage
1 quantity Asian Slaw (see page 82)
½ bunch radishes, trimmed, scrubbed and sliced into thin rounds
2 tablespoons fried shallots

1 Preheat the oven to 180°C and line a baking tray with baking paper.

2 Working with one sheet at a time, spray the filo with cooking oil. Place ¼ of the san choi bao mixture along the short end of the filo sheet, leaving a 5 cm border. Fold the long edges over, then roll to enclose. Spray with cooking oil and place on the prepared tray. Repeat with remaining filo and san choi bao, then bake for 20–25 minutes.

3 Meanwhile, make the Asian slaw and mix with the radish, then sprinkle with fried shallots.

4 Cut each roll into three and serve with the slaw.

# Spiced pork and vermicelli salad ›

**SERVES** 4  PREP **15 mins**  COOK **5 mins**

Light and fresh and with minimal cooking involved, this is a delicious salad to have for lunch.

2 cups (350 g) cooked rice vermicelli noodles
1 quantity Nam Jim Dressing (see page 206)
handful mixed fresh herbs such as mint, coriander and basil
2 carrots, cut into thin matchsticks or coarsely grated
2 Lebanese (small) cucumbers, cut into thin matchsticks
4 spring onions, trimmed and finely sliced
1 × 250 g punnet cherry tomatoes, quartered
75 g iceberg lettuce, shredded
½ quantity (400 g) Spiced Pork Meatballs (see page 82)
½ cup (45 g) Pickled Radish (see page 201) or sliced fresh radish
4 tablespoons fried shallots
1 long red chilli, seeded and finely sliced (optional)

1 Toss the noodles with 1 tablespoon of the dressing and half the herbs and divide among four bowls. Place the carrot, cucumber, spring onion and tomato in a bowl and combine, then mix the remaining dressing through.

2 Layer the lettuce on top of the noodles, then top with the dressed vegetables. Divide the meatballs among the bowls, then scatter over the radish, fried shallots and remaining herbs. Serve the chilli to the side, if using.

**Tip:** Double the amount of pork for 2 units protein.

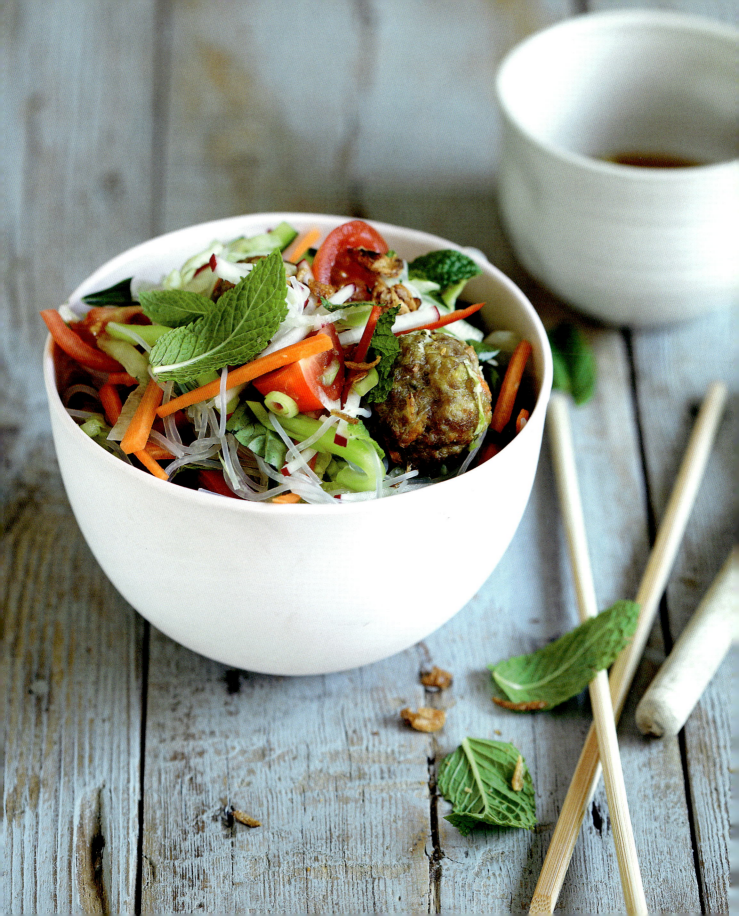

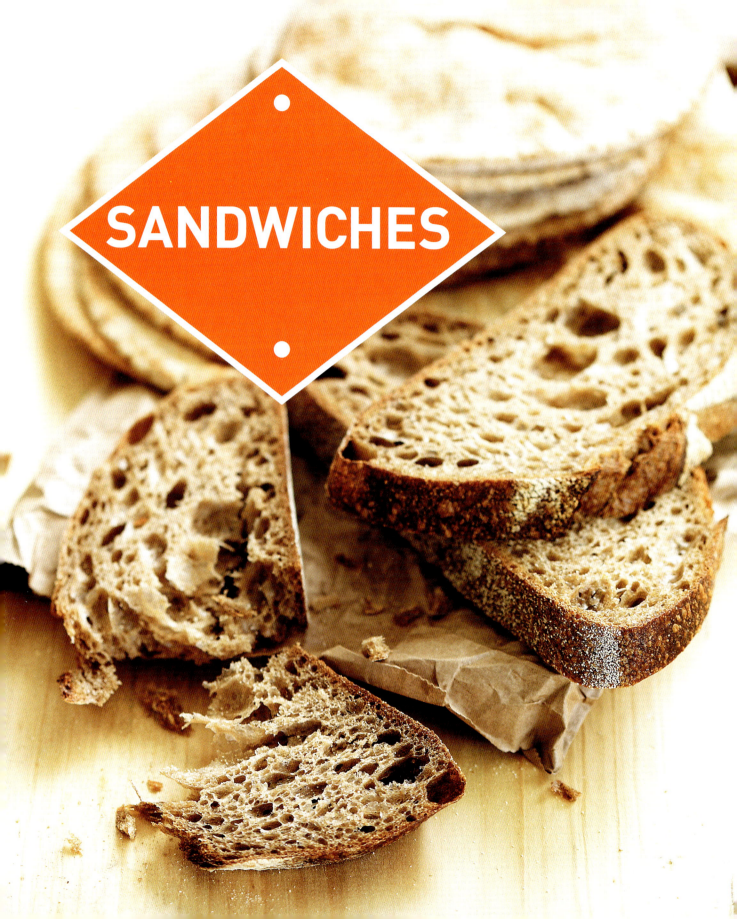

SANDWICHES

# Deluxe chicken sandwiches

MAKES 4  PREP **15 mins**

**The herby lemon flavour of this chicken teams perfectly with zucchini hummus and fresh tomato (or you could use any cooked chicken you have on hand for this).**

400 g shredded chicken from Chicken Baked in a Bread
   Crust (see page 110), mixed with 1½ tablespoons
   cooking juices from the chicken or water
8 slices wholemeal sourdough bread
2 tomatoes, sliced
1 Lebanese (small) cucumber, thinly sliced lengthways
8 pitted green olives, chopped
8 baby cos lettuce leaves
8 tablespoons Zucchini Hummus (see page 204)

1 Divide the chicken among four slices of the bread,
and top with tomato, cucumber, olives and lettuce
leaves. Spread the zucchini hummus on the
remaining slices, season with pepper and place
on top of the sandwich.

# Chicken tikka wraps

MAKES 4  PREP **15 mins**

**Balance is essential in a great wrap. Tossing the cabbage in yoghurt first helps to soften it and ensures the flavours get evenly distributed. Warm the chicken before adding to the wrap, and throw in some fresh coriander if you like.**

160 g reduced-fat plain yoghurt
1 small clove garlic, very finely chopped
1 tablespoon lemon juice
¾ teaspoon ground coriander
2 cups (150 g) finely shredded red cabbage
4 wholemeal wraps, warmed
1 carrot, grated
1 Lebanese (small) cucumber, thinly sliced lengthways
400 g shredded Chicken Tikka (see page 98), warmed

1 Combine the yoghurt, garlic, lemon juice and
coriander in a small bowl, then season to taste
with salt and pepper. Spoon half the yoghurt into
a large bowl, add the cabbage and toss to coat.

2 Divide the cabbage among the wraps, then top
with carrot, cucumber and chicken. Drizzle over
the remaining yoghurt and roll to enclose.

**Tip:** Add 1 teaspoon salt-reduced tomato paste (puree)
to the yoghurt mixture or some freshly sliced tomato.

# Roast beef sandwiches with beetroot and pickled radish

MAKES 4  PREP 15 mins

Use leftovers from the roast beef recipe, or any other cooked beef you have to hand. You could use ready-made low-fat beetroot dip if you don't have time to make your own.

8 tablespoons Roast Beetroot Dip (see page 204)
4 slices wholemeal sourdough bread
400 g sliced Roast Beef (see page 74)
2 tomatoes, sliced
3 tablespoons Pickled Radish (see page 201)
   or sliced fresh radish
50 g feta
8 cos or iceberg lettuce leaves

1 Spread the beetroot dip on the bread slices and top with beef, tomato, radish and feta. Season to taste with salt and pepper and top with lettuce.

# Lamb souvlakis with pickled cucumber

MAKES 4  PREP 15 mins

This healthy version of classic takeaway food is every bit as good, if not better, than the original. Use leftovers from the braised lamb shoulder recipe, or any cooked lamb.

⅔ cup (190 g) reduced-fat plain yoghurt
1 small clove garlic, very finely chopped
1 tablespoon lemon juice
4 pita breads, warmed
400 g shredded Braised Lamb Shoulder
   (see page 84), gently warmed
12 slices Pickled Cucumber (see page 201)
2 tomatoes, sliced
6–8 iceberg lettuce leaves, shredded

1 Combine the yoghurt, garlic and lemon juice in a small bowl and season to taste.

2 Spread 1 tablespoon of the yoghurt mixture on each pita bread, then top with the lamb, cucumber, tomato and lettuce. Drizzle over the remaining yoghurt mixture and roll to enclose.

Tip: For extra flavour, add a few slices of the roast fennel from the braised lamb recipe to each souvlaki.

# Shredded pork and pickled carrot sandwiches

MAKES 4 PREP **10 mins**

The spiced pork and pickled carrot combine to make a delicious sandwich; you can use any leftover cooked pork though.

400 g shredded Cajun-spiced Pork (see page 64)
8 slices wholemeal bread
1 cup (90 g) Pickled Carrot (see page 201)
1 cup (75 g) finely shredded red cabbage
2 tablespoons finely chopped flat-leaf parsley
4 tablespoons labna (see page 28)
pickled jalapeno chillies (optional), to serve

1 Divide the pork among four slices of bread.

2 Combine the carrot, cabbage and parsley, season to taste with salt and pepper, then pile on top of the pork.

3 Spread the labna on the remaining bread slices, and serve with jalapenos, if using.

# Indian-spiced chicken wraps

MAKES 4 PREP **10 mins**

Leftover roast chicken tastes great the next day in a sandwich or wrap: this one features Indian-spiced roast chicken. Use low-fat baba ghanoush if you don't have any eggplant dip on hand.

8 tablespoons Spiced Eggplant Dip (see page 202)
4 wholemeal wraps
400 g shredded Indian-spiced Roast Chicken
  (see page 102)
1 cup (150 g) Pickled Zucchini (see page 201)
½ red (Spanish) onion, thinly sliced
2 large handfuls picked watercress leaves
4 tablespoons reduced-fat plain yoghurt

1 Spread 2 tablespoons eggplant dip on each wrap, then top with the chicken, zucchini, onion and watercress.

2 Top each wrap with 1 tablespoon yoghurt, season to taste with salt and pepper and roll to enclose.

# VEGETABLES, SALADS & SOUPS

# Braised Asian vegetables

SERVES 4  PREP **10 mins**  COOK **5 mins**

2 tablespoons oyster sauce

1½ tablespoons finely
   shredded ginger

3 teaspoons salt-reduced soy sauce

¼ teaspoon sesame oil

½ cup (125 ml) Vegetable Stock
   (see page 209) or water

1 bunch (about 350 g) Chinese broccoli
   (gai lan), trimmed, leaves and
   stems separated

150 g sugar snap peas or snowpeas
   (mange-tout), strings removed

150 g green beans, trimmed

3 spring onions, trimmed and sliced

1 long red chilli, seeded and
   finely sliced

**A great use of a free list vegetable, this is a quick and easy one-pot dish. Serve as a side dish with a curry, or with pan-fried fish, chicken or pork.**

1 Place the oyster sauce, ginger, soy sauce, sesame oil and vegetable stock or water in a large saucepan with a pinch of white pepper. Bring to the boil, then add the Chinese broccoli stems, sugar snaps or snowpeas, green beans and ¾ of the spring onion and chilli. Cover and cook for 3 minutes. Add the Chinese broccoli leaves and cook for a further 1–2 minutes until the vegetables are tender.

2 Using tongs, arrange the vegetables on a warmed plate and drizzle with some of the braising liquid. Scatter with the remaining spring onion and chilli and serve.

**Tip:** Use any vegetables you have to hand, such as carrots, zucchini or broccoli, cut into similar-sized pieces.

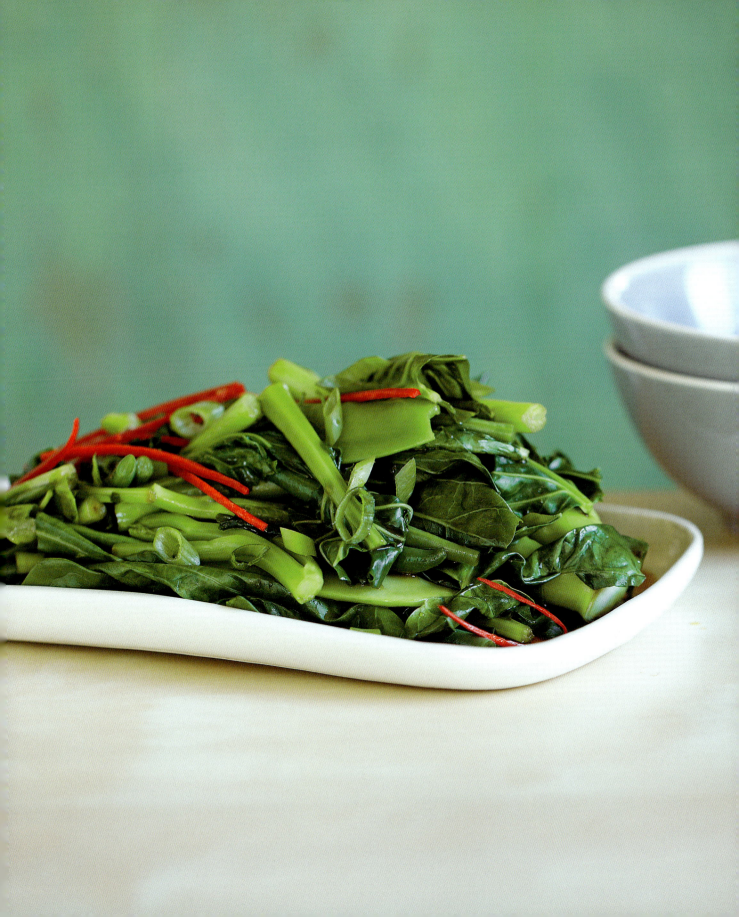

1 SERVE =
**2½ units vegetables**
**1½ units fats**

# Middle Eastern-spiced ratatouille

SERVES 4  PREP **15 mins**  COOK **1 hour**

1 tablespoon olive oil

1 red (Spanish) onion, sliced

1 red capsicum (pepper),
  trimmed, seeded and chopped
  into 3 cm pieces

1 green capsicum (pepper),
  trimmed, seeded, and chopped
  into 3 cm pieces

2 eggplants (aubergines),
  cut into 3 cm cubes

cooking oil spray

2 tomatoes, roughly chopped

1 tablespoon ground coriander

3 teaspoons ground sumac

½ teaspoon ground allspice

2 zucchinis (courgettes), trimmed
  and chopped into 3 cm pieces

3 cloves garlic, finely chopped

2 teaspoons sesame seeds

**Middle Eastern spices turn this French classic into the perfect accompaniment to just about any meal. If you grow your own herbs, stir through some chopped fresh mint, coriander or flat-leaf parsley at the end to make this dish extra special.**

1 Place a large saucepan over medium–high heat. Add the olive oil and onion and cook for 3–4 minutes until the onion begins to soften. Add the red and green capsicum and cook for 2 minutes. Spray the eggplant with cooking oil, then add to the pan and cook, stirring, for 5 minutes until the eggplant begins to soften. Add the tomato and ground spices, then reduce the heat to low and cook, covered, for 30 minutes, stirring occasionally. Add the zucchini and garlic, season to taste with salt and pepper and cook, covered, for 20 minutes until all the vegetables are very tender.

2 Meanwhile, toast the sesame seeds in a dry frying pan over medium heat for 3–4 minutes until lightly golden. Set aside.

3 Serve the ratatouille sprinkled with toasted sesame seeds.

**Tip:** Add 1⅓ cups (250 g) drained tinned chickpeas for 1 bread unit.

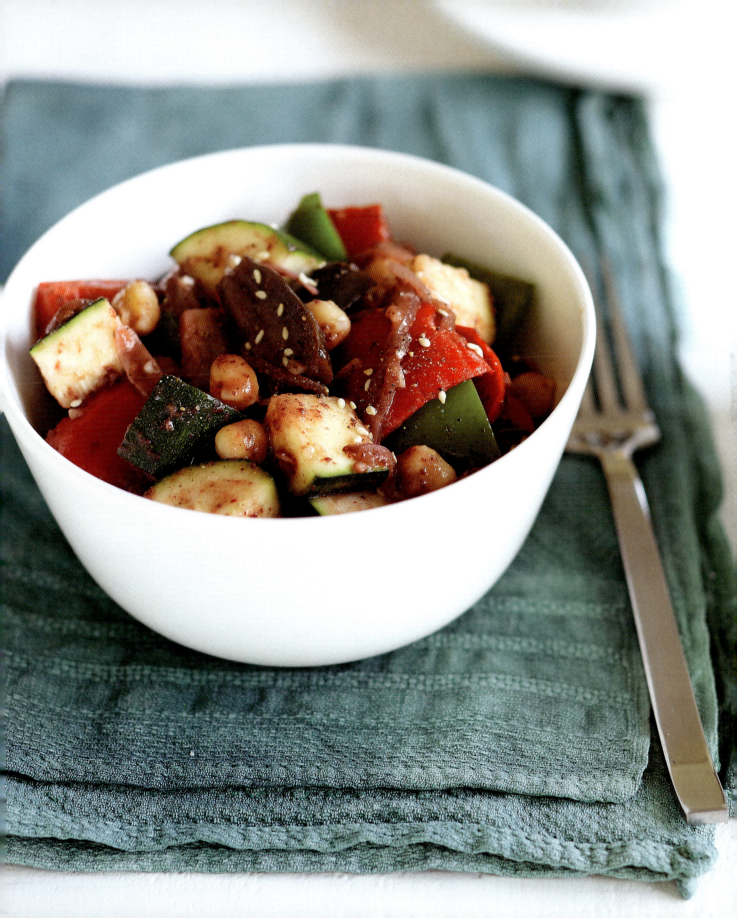

# Braised green beans with tomato and oregano

SERVES 4  PREP **10 mins**  COOK **35 mins**

**A great side dish to have with pan-fried chicken, pork or fish. Cook the beans until they are soft but still holding their shape.**

1 tablespoon olive oil
½ onion, finely sliced
2 cloves garlic, sliced
1 teaspoon dried oregano
1 × 400 g tin peeled tomatoes
2 teaspoons salt-reduced tomato paste (puree)
450 g green beans, trimmed

1 Place a large saucepan over medium heat. Add the olive oil, onion, garlic and oregano and cook for 3–4 minutes until the onion begins to soften. Add the tomato, tomato paste and beans, season to taste with salt and pepper and stir to combine. Bring to simmering point then reduce the heat to low, cover and cook for 20 minutes. Remove the lid and cook for a further 5–10 minutes until the beans are soft and tender but not falling apart.

**Tip:** Try adding a pinch of chilli flakes or cayenne pepper for some extra kick, or sprinkle the beans with 50 g reduced-fat feta for ¼ dairy unit.

# Honey-roasted carrots with cumin and caraway ›

SERVES 4  PREP **10 mins**  COOK **50 mins**

**Cumin and caraway are the perfect partners to caramelised roasted carrots.**

600 g carrots, peeled, trimmed and
    quartered lengthways
1 teaspoon cumin seeds
1 teaspoon caraway seeds
2 teaspoons honey, warmed
cooking oil spray

1 Preheat the oven to 200°C and line a baking tray with baking paper.
2 Combine the carrot, spices and honey in a large bowl. Spray with oil, season to taste with salt and pepper and toss to coat. Arrange the carrot in a single layer on the prepared tray, then roast for 45–50 minutes until golden and tender.

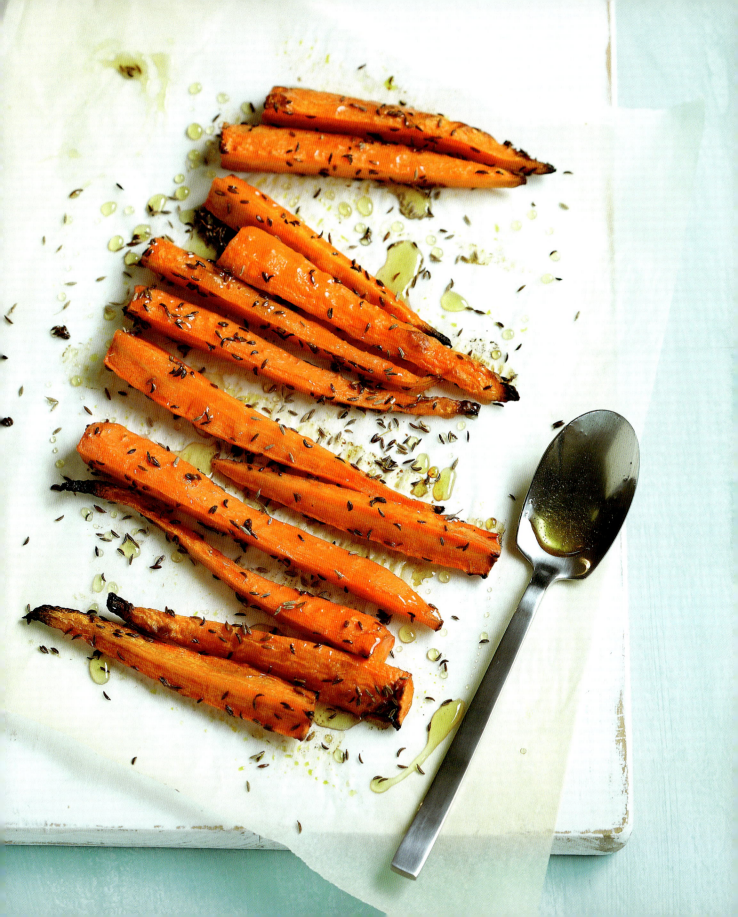

# Garlic and mint pea puree

SERVES 4  PREP **5 mins**  COOK **5 mins**

**Mint and green peas were made for each other. Combined with garlic and a dollop of yoghurt, this puree is good enough to eat on its own.**

2 cloves garlic, sliced
3 cups (360 g) frozen peas
2 tablespoons reduced-fat plain yoghurt
1 tablespoon chopped mint or 1 teaspoon dried mint

1 Bring a saucepan of water to the boil and add the garlic. Cook for 1 minute, then add the peas and cook for a further 2 minutes, then drain.

2 Combine the peas, garlic, yoghurt and mint in the bowl of a food processor and blend until smooth. Season to taste with salt and pepper and serve.

# Carrot puree

SERVES 4  PREP **10 mins**  COOK **15 mins**

**Use this puree to dress up roast chicken, to sweeten barbecued pork or to add a splash of colour to slow-roasted lamb.**

450 g carrots, peeled, trimmed and chopped
2 teaspoons honey
½ teaspoon red wine vinegar
¼ teaspoon ground cumin or ginger

1 Place the carrot in a saucepan along with enough water to barely cover it. Bring to the boil, then cover, reduce the heat and simmer for 15 minutes until tender. Drain, reserving about 1½ tablespoons of the cooking liquid.

2 Place the carrot in the bowl of a food processor with the remaining ingredients and 1 tablespoon of the reserved cooking liquid. Process until smooth, adding more cooking liquid if necessary. Season to taste with salt and pepper and serve.

# Parsnip and cauliflower puree

SERVES 4–6  PREP **10 mins**  COOK **20 mins**

**Parsnips and cauliflower are a great combination – here the starch in the parsnips helps to bind the puree. This is an excellent alternative to mashed potato.**

300 g parsnips, peeled and cut into 3 cm chunks
300 g cauliflower, cut into florets
4 cloves garlic, peeled
2 teaspoons horseradish cream
1–2 tablespoons reduced-fat milk

1 Bring a large saucepan of water to the boil, add the parsnips and simmer gently for 10 minutes. Add the cauliflower and garlic and cook for a further 10 minutes until the vegetables are tender, then drain well.

2 Place the vegetables in the bowl of a food processor with the horseradish cream and 1 tablespoon milk and season to taste with salt and pepper. Process until smooth, adding more milk if necessary. Serve immediately.

**Tip:** If you don't have a food processor, simply mash the vegetables by hand, gradually mixing in the horseradish cream and milk until you have a rough puree. Stir through some chopped chives or flat-leaf parsley for a fresh note.

# Pumpkin and sweet potato mash

SERVES 4  PREP **10 mins**  COOK **30 mins**

**Low in carbs, this rustic mash isn't as smooth as mashed potato, but the smoky sweet flavour of the spiced roast vegetables will delight. Serve with any hearty stew or braise.**

300 g pumpkin (squash), trimmed, peeled and cut into 2 cm pieces
300 g sweet potato, peeled and cut into 2 cm pieces
4 cloves garlic, peeled and halved
cooking oil spray
½ teaspoon sweet paprika
½ teaspoon ground cumin
2 tablespoons reduced-fat milk

1 Preheat the oven to 220°C and line a baking tray with baking paper.

2 Spread out the vegetables on the prepared tray, spray with cooking oil and season with salt and pepper to taste. Sprinkle over the ground spices and roast for 25–30 minutes, turning once, until tender and golden.

3 Transfer the vegetables to a large bowl, add the milk and roughly mash, adding more milk if the mixture is too dry. Serve immediately.

# Braised red cabbage with honey and mustard

SERVES 4 PREP **10 mins** COOK **20 mins**

¾ red cabbage (600 g), cored
  and finely shredded
1 onion, finely sliced
2 cloves garlic, finely sliced
2 tablespoons apple cider
  vinegar or red wine vinegar
1 tablespoon
  wholegrain mustard
3 teaspoons honey

**Braising cabbage releases a natural sweetness that teams beautifully with mustard and honey. Serve with roast chicken or pork, barbecued meats or vegie burgers.**

1 Combine all the ingredients and 2 tablespoons water in a medium-sized saucepan, season to taste with salt and pepper and stir to combine. Cover and cook over low heat, stirring occasionally, for 12–15 minutes until the cabbage is soft but still retains some bite.

2 Remove the lid and cook for 3–4 minutes until most of the liquid has evaporated. Serve immediately.

**Tip:** Add some chopped fresh herbs, such as flat-leaf parsley, chives or dill, and a squeeze of lemon juice before serving.

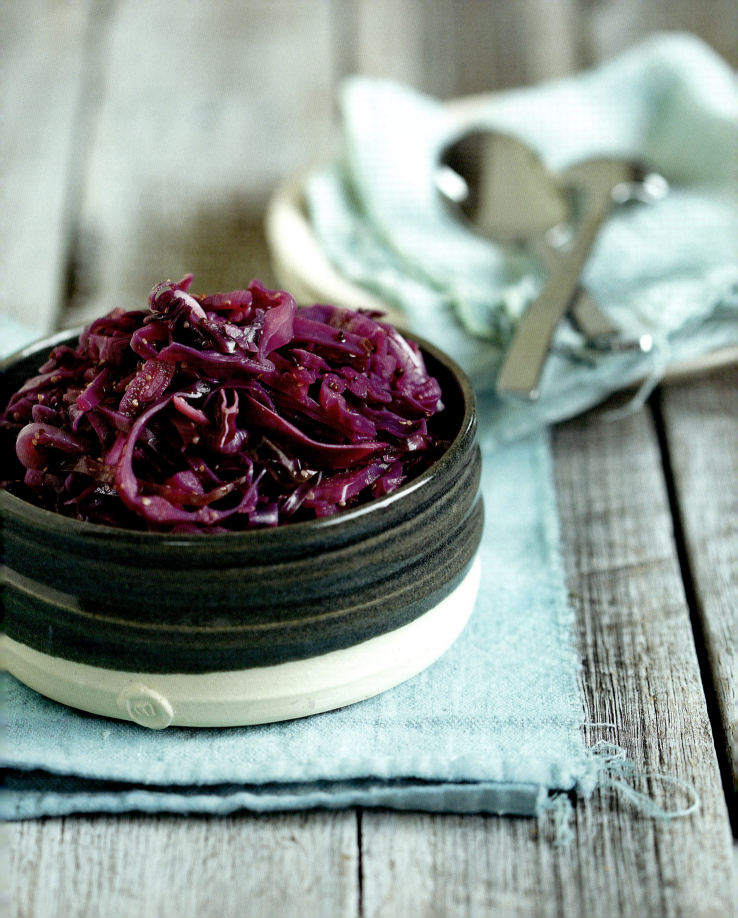

375 g broccoli, roughly chopped
1 cup (120 g) frozen peas
1 tablespoon light margarine
½ red (Spanish) onion, finely diced
2 cloves garlic, crushed
½ teaspoon ground sumac
1 tablespoon lemon juice
1 tablespoon chopped flat-leaf
   parsley (optional)

# Sumac-spiced broccoli and peas

SERVES 4  PREP **10 mins**  COOK **10 mins**

**Fresh, zesty and subtly sweet, this dish works well as a side with just about any protein. Cook the broccoli until it is tender but not mushy, as you want to retain as much of the nutrition as possible.**

1 Bring a large saucepan of water to the boil and add the broccoli. Boil for 5 minutes until tender, adding the peas for the last minute of cooking time, then drain well.

2 Meanwhile, place a large frying pan over medium–high heat. Add the margarine, onion, garlic and sumac and cook for 7–8 minutes until the onion is soft, then reduce the heat to low. Add the vegetables and lemon juice, season to taste with salt and pepper and serve immediately.

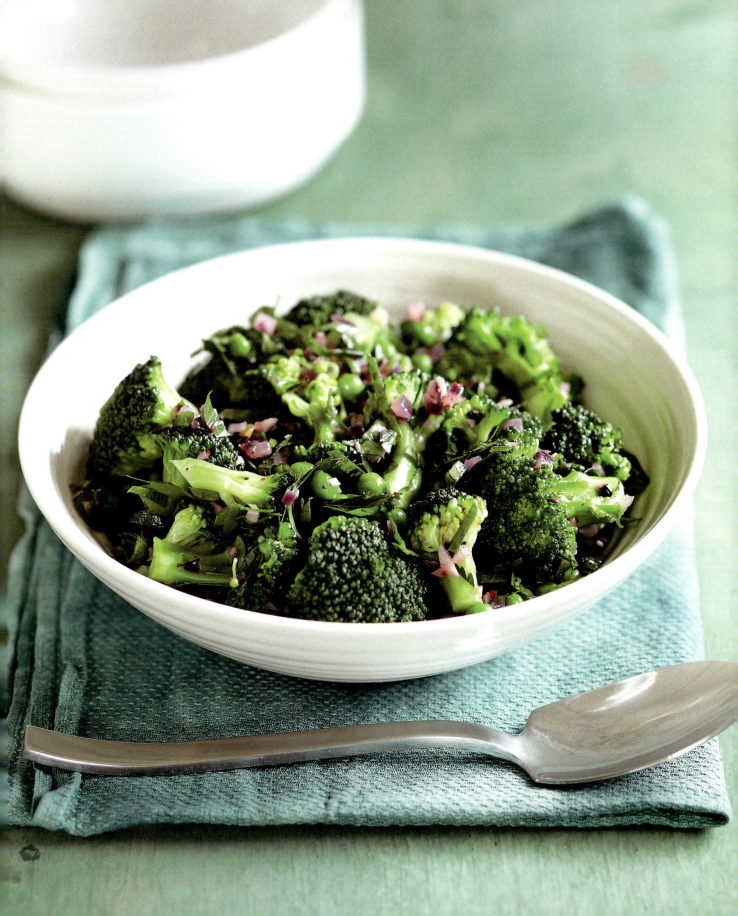

3 capsicums (peppers), trimmed,
    seeded and quartered
3 medium-sized tomatoes
1½ tablespoons red wine vinegar
1 tablespoon extra virgin olive oil
1 clove garlic, crushed
2 teaspoons oregano leaves,
    roughly chopped or ½ teaspoon
    dried oregano
2 tablespoon drained capers

# Roast capsicum and tomato salad

SERVES 4  PREP **15 mins, plus standing time**  COOK **10 mins**

**Combining smoky roast capsicum with sweet fresh tomatoes, this simple salad only gets better the longer it sits. Prepare it an hour or two in advance to allow time for the flavours to combine.**

1 Place the capsicum, skin-side up, under a grill in a single layer and cook for 8–10 minutes until the skins blacken and blister. Transfer to a bowl, cover with plastic wrap and leave to stand for 10 minutes to steam (this will help loosen the skins). Remove the plastic, peel away the skins and discard. Slice the capsicum into 2 cm thick slices.

2 Cut a cross in the bottom of each tomato and place in a deep bowl. Cover with boiling water and leave for 45 seconds before removing with a slotted spoon. When cool enough to handle, remove the skins, scoop out the seeds and slice the flesh into 2 cm wedges.

3 Place the tomato in a bowl with the roast capsicum, vinegar, olive oil, garlic and oregano. Season to taste with salt and pepper and toss gently to combine. Leave to stand at room temperature for 30–60 minutes to allow the flavours to infuse. Sprinkle over the capers just before serving.

Tip: Add some chopped flat-leaf parsley, a pinch of smoked paprika or the finely grated zest of ½ lemon for extra zing.

# Green salad

SERVES 4 PREP **15 mins**

This simple salad combines the crunch of snowpeas, the creaminess of raw zucchini and the sweetness of cherry tomatoes to great effect. Add some fresh mixed herbs from the garden for that extra lift. Use any salad vegetables you have on hand (or try adding some finely shredded raw pumpkin – it's delicious!).

4 cups (160 g) torn mixed lettuce leaves (such as red
   leaf, cos, butter, watercress, rocket, curly endive)
150 g snowpeas (mange-tout),
   finely shredded lengthways
1 zucchini (courgette), sliced into fine rounds
1 × 250 g punnet cherry tomatoes, halved
1 quantity Herb Dressing (see page 206)

1 Fill a large bowl with cold water and gently submerge the lettuce leaves. Drain in a colander for a couple of minutes, then spin dry in batches.

2 Combine the lettuce leaves with the shredded snowpeas, zucchini and tomato, season with salt and pepper and toss the dressing through. Serve immediately.

**Tip:** If you want to save a fat unit, simply dress the salad with a splash of red wine, balsamic, sherry or apple cider vinegar, or a generous squeeze of lemon or orange juice.

# Tomato and onion salad

SERVES 4 PREP **10 mins, plus standing time**

Raw onion can have an intense taste, but soaking it in cold water mellows the flavour considerably and stops it overpowering the other ingredients.

½ small red (Spanish) onion, halved, thinly sliced
1 tablespoon extra virgin olive oil
1 clove garlic, crushed
1 tablespoon sherry vinegar or red wine vinegar
600 g tomatoes, sliced into 5 mm thick rounds
½ teaspoon smoked paprika

1 Place the onion in a bowl and cover with cold water. Set aside for 15 minutes, then drain well.

2 Combine the olive oil, garlic and vinegar and mix well.

3 Arrange the tomato slices on a large plate, sprinkle with the smoked paprika and season with salt and pepper. Arrange the onion slices on top of the tomato, then drizzle with the dressing. Leave to stand at room temperature for 30 minutes to allow the flavours to develop.

# Shaved cabbage, radish and fennel salad

**SERVES 4** PREP **15 mins**

Serve this low-fat, refreshing salad alongside roast chicken or fish, barbecue pork or to fill sandwiches when going on a picnic. Use Pickled Radish (see page 201) instead of fresh if you have some on hand.

3 cups (225 g) thinly sliced cabbage
1 carrot, finely shredded or coarsely grated
1 bunch radishes, trimmed, scrubbed and
   sliced into thin rounds
1 small bulb fennel, trimmed and finely sliced,
   fronds reserved
3 sticks celery, finely sliced lengthways
4 spring onions, trimmed and finely sliced
handful mint leaves, torn
1 quantity Salad Cream (see page 207)

1 Combine all the ingredients (except the fennel fronds) in a large bowl, then season to taste with salt and pepper and toss gently to combine. Divide among bowls and top with the reserved fennel fronds.

**Tip:** Serve with either 25 g toasted pine nuts (adds 1 fat unit), 40 g shaved parmesan (adds ½ dairy unit) or 2 slices sourdough bread, baked in a preheated 180°C oven for 10 minutes until crisp (adds ½ bread unit).

# Beetroot, carrot and radish salad ›

**SERVES 4** PREP **15 mins**

A great way to use raw beetroot, this fresh and vibrant salad is quick to prepare and packed with nutrients. Serve with barbecued lamb, beef or sausages.

2 large beetroot, peeled and shredded
   or coarsely grated
2 carrots, shredded or coarsely grated
½ bunch radishes, trimmed, scrubbed
   and coarsely grated
2 baby cos lettuces, leaves separated and torn
small handful flat-leaf parsley or
   mint leaves, chopped
3 teaspoons sesame seeds, toasted

**CREAMY CUMIN DRESSING**
4 tablespoons reduced-fat plain yoghurt
1 tablespoon white balsamic vinegar
pinch ground cumin

1 For the dressing, combine all the ingredients with 2 teaspoons water in a large bowl and season to taste with salt and pepper.

2 Add the beetroot, carrot, radish, lettuce and herbs to the dressing and toss to coat. Divide among four bowls and sprinkle with sesame seeds to serve.

**Tip:** To give this salad a sweet touch, serve with 1 coarsely grated green apple or 2 tablespoons chopped raisins (adds 1 fruit unit). Alternatively, serve with 2 tablespoons chopped roasted walnuts for 1 fat unit.

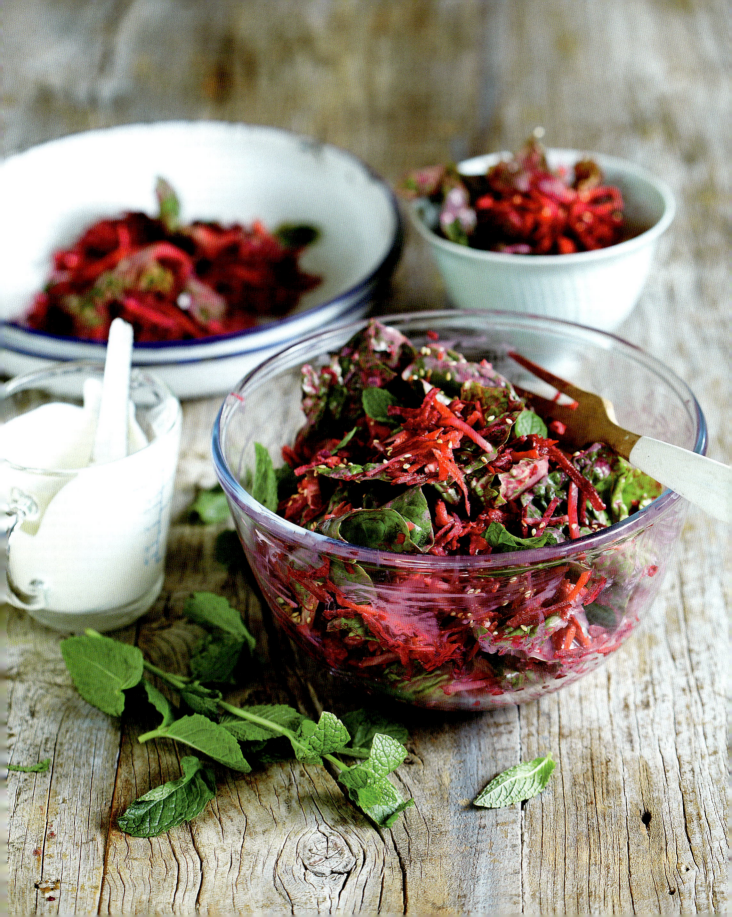

# Warm zucchini and green bean salad with lemon and sumac

**SERVES 4** PREP **15 mins** COOK **15 mins**

2 lemons, peeled and pith removed

3 corn cobs

4 zucchinis (courgettes), cut on the
   diagonal into 3 cm thick slices

1 carrot, sliced into 1 cm rounds

75 g green beans, trimmed

80 g baby spinach leaves

large handful flat-leaf parsley
   or mint leaves

**DRESSING**

1 tablespoon olive oil

1 clove garlic, crushed

1–2 teaspoons ground sumac

2 tablespoons white balsamic vinegar

**This fresh and zesty warm vegetable salad is a wonderful accompaniment, or you could add some cooked couscous or pearl barley to make it a meal in itself. For ½ a protein unit add 2 soft-boiled eggs to each serve.**

1 Segment the lemons by holding them over a bowl and using a small, sharp knife to cut the flesh away from the inner membrane, letting the juice drop into the bowl. Slice each segment in half lengthways, then add to the bowl and set aside.

2 For the dressing, combine all the ingredients and set aside to allow the flavours to infuse.

3 Bring a large saucepan of water to the boil, add the corn and cook for 10 minutes until tender. Remove with tongs then, when cool enough to handle, place the cobs on their ends and carefully slice off the kernels.

4 Steam the zucchini, carrot and green beans for 5 minutes until tender, adding the corn for the last minute to reheat. Transfer the vegetables and spinach to a large bowl, drizzle over the dressing and season to taste with salt and pepper. Toss through the lemon segments and parsley or mint and serve.

**Tip:** Try this with 20 g chopped pitted green olives per serve for 1 extra fat unit.

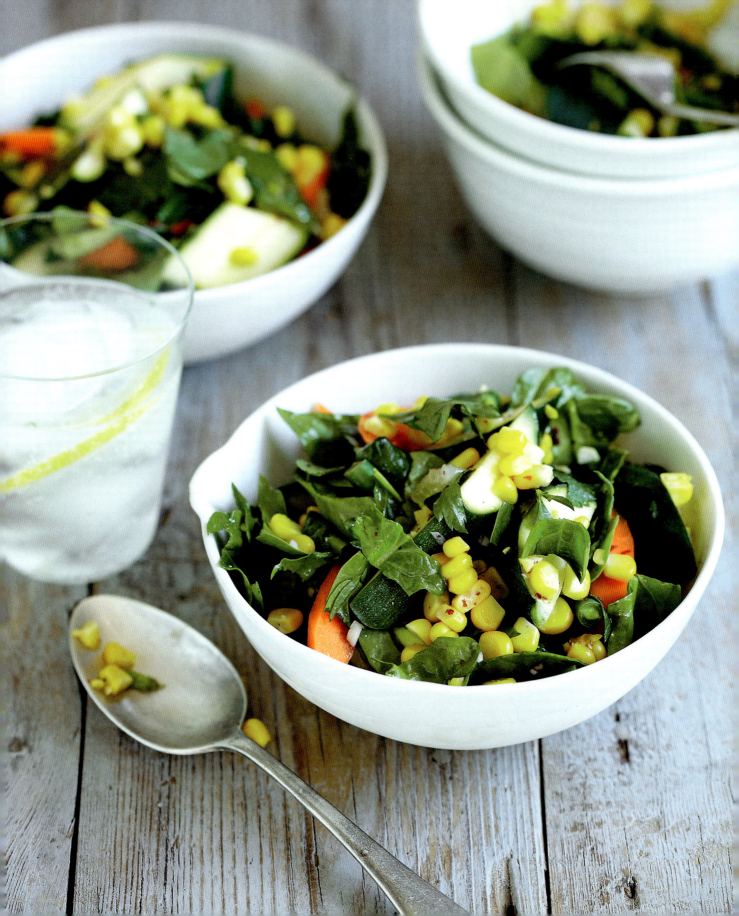

1 SERVE =
½ unit bread
¼ unit dairy
1½ units vegetables

# Roast pumpkin and zucchini salad with blackened corn

SERVES 4  PREP **15 mins, plus cooling time**  COOK **30 mins**

450 g pumpkin (squash), unpeeled,
    seeded and sliced into 1 cm wedges
2 red (Spanish) onions, sliced into
    1 cm thick rings
2 zucchinis (courgettes), sliced into
    1.5 cm thick rounds
cooking oil spray
1 tablespoon fresh thyme leaves
    or 2 teaspoons dried thyme
1 corn cob
4 tablespoons reduced-fat
    Greek-style yoghurt
2 tablespoons red wine vinegar
few drops Tabasco sauce
1 × 250 g punnet cherry
    tomatoes, halved
120 g rocket leaves

**Cook the vegetables until they start to darken around the edges to give this hearty salad a delicious smoky flavour.**

1 Preheat the oven to 220°C and line a baking tray with baking paper.

2 Arrange the pumpkin, onion and zucchini on the prepared tray and spray with cooking oil. Season to taste with salt and pepper, then scatter with thyme. Roast the vegetables for 25–30 minutes, turning once, until golden and tender. Remove from the oven and allow to cool for 10 minutes.

3 Meanwhile, heat a barbecue or chargrill pan to high and cook the corn, turning often, for 6–8 minutes until slightly charred and tender. When cool enough to handle, place the cob on its end and carefully slice off the kernels, then add to the roast vegetables.

4 Combine the yoghurt, vinegar, Tabasco and 1 tablespoon cold water in a small bowl. Season to taste with salt and pepper, then mix well to combine. Place the tomato and rocket in a small bowl, drizzle over half the dressing and toss to combine.

5 Spoon the tomato and rocket mixture onto a serving platter. Arrange the vegetables on top, then drizzle over the remaining dressing and serve.

**Tip:** Serve with 20 g toasted flaked almonds scattered over the platter for ¾ fat unit per serve, or add 1⅓ cups (365 g) cooked white beans to the recipe for 1 bread unit per serve.

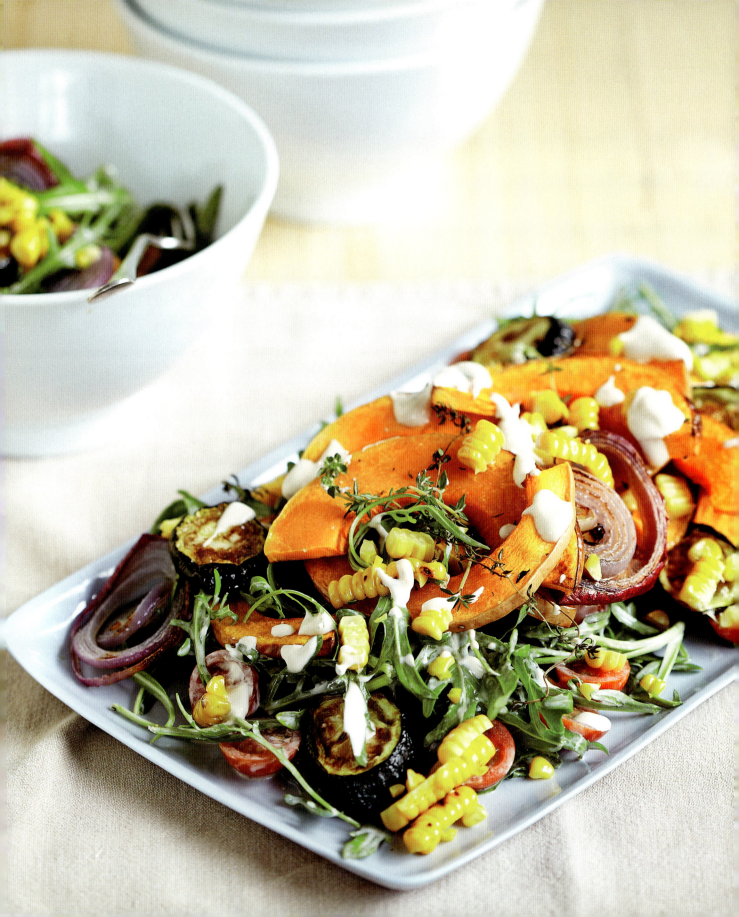

2 eggplants (aubergines),
   halved lengthways
4 cloves garlic, 3 halved, 1 crushed
100 g reduced-fat plain yoghurt
finely grated zest and juice of 1 lemon
½ teaspoon ground sumac
   or ground cumin
½ teaspoon dried mint
chopped coriander and chopped
   green chilli, to serve

# Eggplant, mint and coriander salad

SERVES 4  PREP **10 mins, plus cooling time**  COOK **8 mins**

**Steaming eggplant is a simple way to cook it without using lots of oil, and gives a silky smooth texture. Prepare the yoghurt dressing and eggplant, then mix them together just before serving, as the eggplant will discolour the yoghurt mixture.**

1 Bring a medium-sized saucepan of water to the boil. Place the eggplant and halved garlic cloves in a steamer basket, cover and cook over rapidly boiling water for 7–8 minutes until the eggplant is tender and a skewer easily passes through the flesh. Remove from the heat and set aside to cool.

2 Squash the cooked garlic cloves with the back of a knife to a paste, and place in a bowl with the yoghurt, lemon zest and juice, sumac or cumin, mint and crushed raw garlic. Season to taste with salt and pepper and mix well to combine. When the eggplant is cool, cut it into bite-sized pieces, then mix through the yoghurt dressing, chopped coriander and chilli and serve.

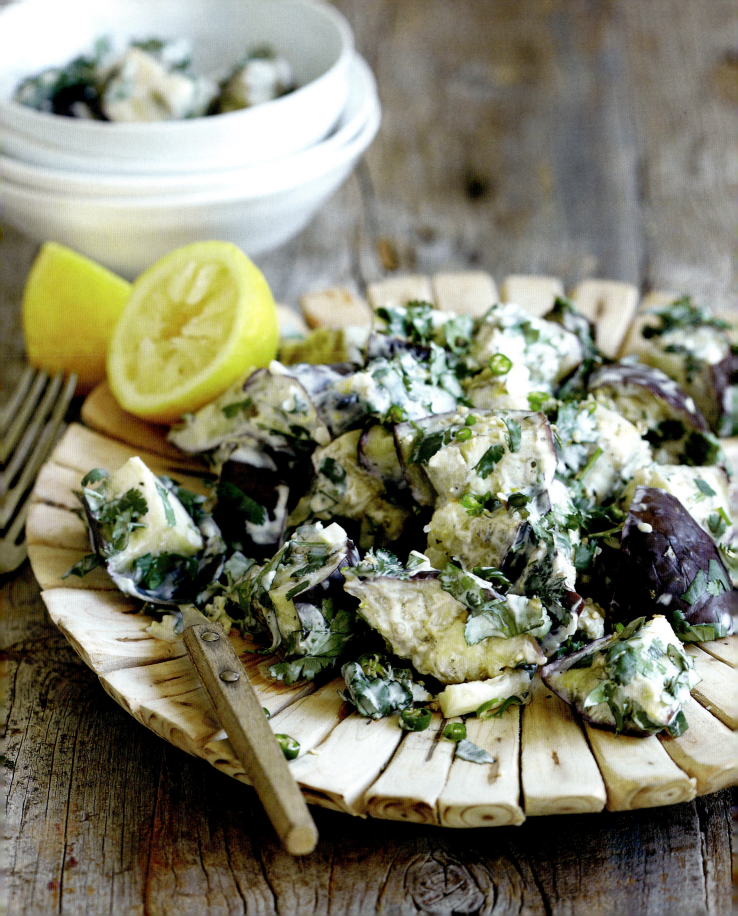

1 SERVE =
½ unit bread
1½ units vegetables
1 unit fats

1 bunch beetroot, trimmed, peeled
   and sliced into 2 cm wedges
300 g sweet potato, peeled and cut
   into 3 cm pieces
1 carrot, cut on the diagonal into
   5 mm thick rounds
2 red (Spanish) onions,
   cut into 2 cm wedges
1 head garlic,
   cloves separated, unpeeled
cooking oil spray
2 sprigs rosemary, leaves stripped
   or 2 teaspoons dried rosemary
2 teaspoons cumin seeds
1 quantity Salsa Verde (see page 207),
   to serve
120 g baby spinach leaves
handful mint leaves, to garnish

# Roast vegetable salad with salsa verde

SERVES 4  PREP **20 mins**  COOK **1 hour**

**This wholesome salad perfectly balances the natural sweetness of roast veggies with a zesty salsa verde dressing. For a substantial meal, toss with 1⅓ cups (200 g) cooked couscous for 1 bread unit per serve, and add your choice of protein (meat, chicken, fish, eggs or tofu).**

1 Preheat the oven to 220°C.

2 Place the beetroot in a small baking dish, season to taste with salt and pepper and cover with foil. Roast for 30 minutes, then remove the foil and continue to roast for a further 25–30 minutes until tender.

3 Meanwhile, combine the sweet potato, carrot, onion and garlic on baking-paper-lined baking trays, spray with cooking oil and season to taste with salt and pepper. Scatter over the rosemary and cumin seeds, then add to the oven when you remove the foil from the beetroot. Roast for 25–30 minutes until the vegetables are golden and tender.

4 Make the dressing, then squeeze four cloves of garlic from their skins and mix into the dressing.

5 Arrange the roast vegetables and spinach on plates, then drizzle over the dressing and scatter with mint.

Tip: For added crunch, top this salad with 40 g toasted pepitas (adds 1 unit fat).

½ red (Spanish) onion, thinly sliced

3 cloves garlic, chopped

2 teaspoons dried Italian herbs

1 teaspoon fennel seeds

pinch chilli flakes

2 cups (500 ml) unsweetened
    tomato juice

½ cup (125 ml) Chicken Stock
    (see page 209)

1 tablespoon extra virgin olive oil

1 tablespoon red wine vinegar

1.5 kg tomatoes, halved

3–4 teaspoons balsamic vinegar

# Slow-roasted tomato soup

SERVES 4  PREP **20 mins**  COOK **2 hours**

**More than just your everyday tomato soup, this slow-roasted version redefines a much-loved favourite. Slow-roasting intensifies the natural sweetness in the tomatoes, so try to use very ripe, in-season varieties.**

1 Preheat the oven to 150°C.

2 Scatter the onion, garlic, herbs, fennel seeds and chilli flakes in a deep roasting tin that will snugly fit the tomatoes. Combine the tomato juice, stock, olive oil and red wine vinegar and season to taste with salt and pepper. Place the tomatoes, cut-side down, in the tin and pour over the tomato juice. Roast for 2 hours, until the tomatoes are breaking down and the onion is very soft.

3 Remove from the oven and use tongs to gently pull away as much tomato skin as possible (it should slip off very easily), then blend the tomato mixture until smooth using a hand-held blender.

4 Transfer the soup to a saucepan and warm through over medium heat. Stir in the balsamic vinegar to taste, and season with salt and pepper.

5 Spoon the soup into bowls, and serve with bread from your daily allowance if desired.

**Tip:** For a light lunch, serve this soup with 100 g poached white fish per person for 1 unit protein.

# Hearty vegetable soup

SERVES 4  PREP **15 mins**  COOK **30 mins**

1 tablespoon olive oil

1 onion, finely chopped

2 carrots, roughly chopped

300 g pumpkin (squash), peeled and
    roughly chopped

1 tablespoon dried Italian herbs

3 cloves garlic, finely chopped

150 g green beans, trimmed
    and cut into 3 cm lengths

600 g tinned tomatoes

3 cups (750 ml) Chicken Stock
    (see page 209)

2 zucchinis (courgettes), chopped into
    small chunks

small handful flat-leaf
    parsley leaves, chopped

**Taking its cue from traditional minestrone, this pasta-free version is rich and warming. Don't rush the first step, as 'sweating' the vegetables in this way adds greatly to the flavour of the soup. You can use any leftover vegetables that you have in the fridge in this recipe: spinach, corn, celery and cauliflower will all work well.**

1 Place a large heavy-based stockpot over medium heat. Add the olive oil, onion, carrot, pumpkin and dried herbs and cook, stirring occasionally, for 7–8 minutes until the vegetables soften. Add the garlic and cook for 2 minutes. Add the green beans, tomato and stock, season to taste with salt and pepper and bring to the boil. Reduce the heat and simmer for 10 minutes. Add the zucchini and simmer for a further 7–8 minutes until the vegetables are tender. Stir through the parsley and serve.

**Tip:** If you like, stir through 200 g cooked cannellini beans at the end just to warm them through (adds ½ unit bread), and scatter over 50 g grated parmesan (adds ½ unit dairy).

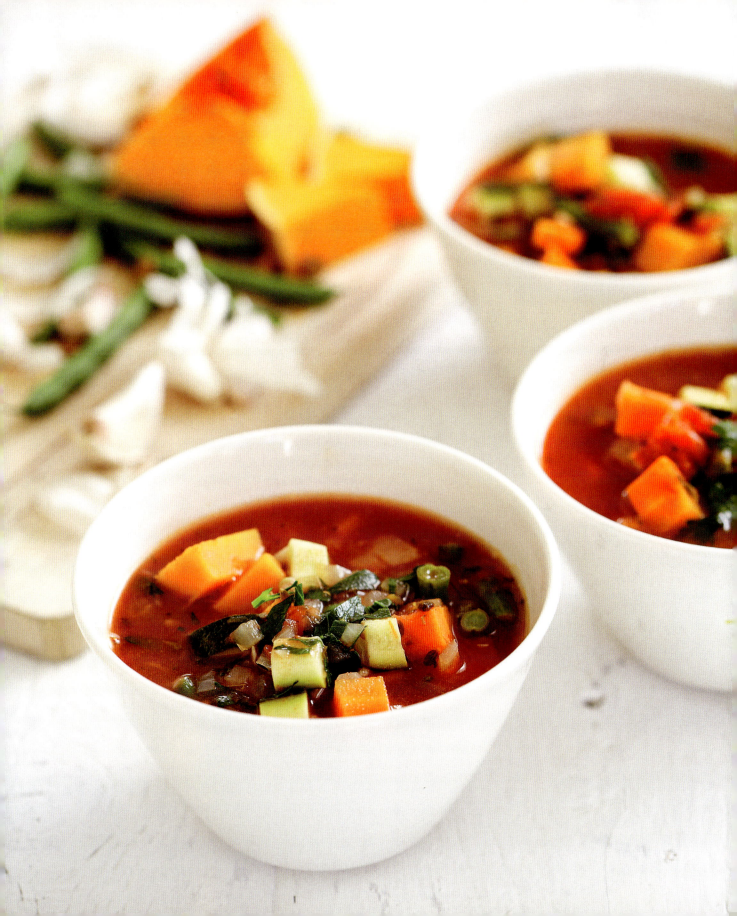

# Asian-scented vegetable broth

SERVES 4  PREP **10 mins**  COOK **20 mins**

**This quick-cooked aromatic soup will soon top your list of favourites, and using homemade chicken stock will only add to the flavour. If you like, add a dash of Chinese chilli sauce or soy sauce just before serving.**

3 teaspoons peanut oil
1½ tablespoons finely shredded ginger
1 long red chilli, seeded and finely sliced
4 spring onions, trimmed and finely sliced,
    white and green parts reserved separately
1.5 litres Chicken Stock (see page 209)
1 tablespoon Chinese Shaohsing rice wine
    or dry cooking sherry
1 tablespoon oyster sauce
1 bunch (300 g) baby bok choy,
    quartered lengthways and washed
1 carrot, cut into matchsticks
150 g snowpeas (mange-tout), trimmed
½–1 teaspoon sesame oil

1 Place a large heavy-based stockpot over medium–high heat. Add the peanut oil, ginger, chilli and the white part of the spring onion and cook for 2 minutes. Add the stock, wine or sherry, oyster sauce and a pinch of white pepper. Bring to the boil, then reduce the heat and simmer for 10 minutes. Add the vegetables and simmer for 4–5 minutes until tender. Season with sesame oil, then ladle into bowls and serve immediately.

**Tip:** To add 1 protein unit, add 400 g diced chicken thigh fillet to the broth after it has come to the boil and poach gently for 10 minutes.

# Coriander and vegetable soup ›

SERVES 4  PREP **15 mins**  COOK **40 mins**

**This is a refreshing, spicy soup – you can omit the chilli from step 1 if you prefer it a little milder.**

1.5 litres salt-reduced ready-made beef stock
1 onion, halved, thinly sliced
1 × 8 cm piece ginger,
    peeled and thinly sliced
10 coriander seeds
4 coriander roots, scraped
4 star anise
1 cinnamon stick
½ long red chilli
2 carrots, sliced into thin rounds
225 g green beans, trimmed
    and cut into 3 cm lengths
1 tablespoon fish sauce

TO SERVE
bean sprouts, coriander and Vietnamese mint leaves, finely sliced long red chilli, lime halves, hoisin sauce and Chinese chilli sauce

1 Place the stock, onion, ginger, coriander seeds and roots, star anise, cinnamon and chilli in a large heavy-based stockpot and bring to the boil. Reduce the heat and simmer for 30 minutes. Remove the spices and discard. Add the carrot, beans and fish sauce and season with black pepper. Cover and simmer for 6–7 minutes until the vegetables are tender.

2 Ladle the soup into bowls and top with the bean sprouts, herbs and chilli. Squeeze over some lime juice and serve the sauces to the side.

**Tip:** Add 400 g sliced roast beef for 1 protein unit.

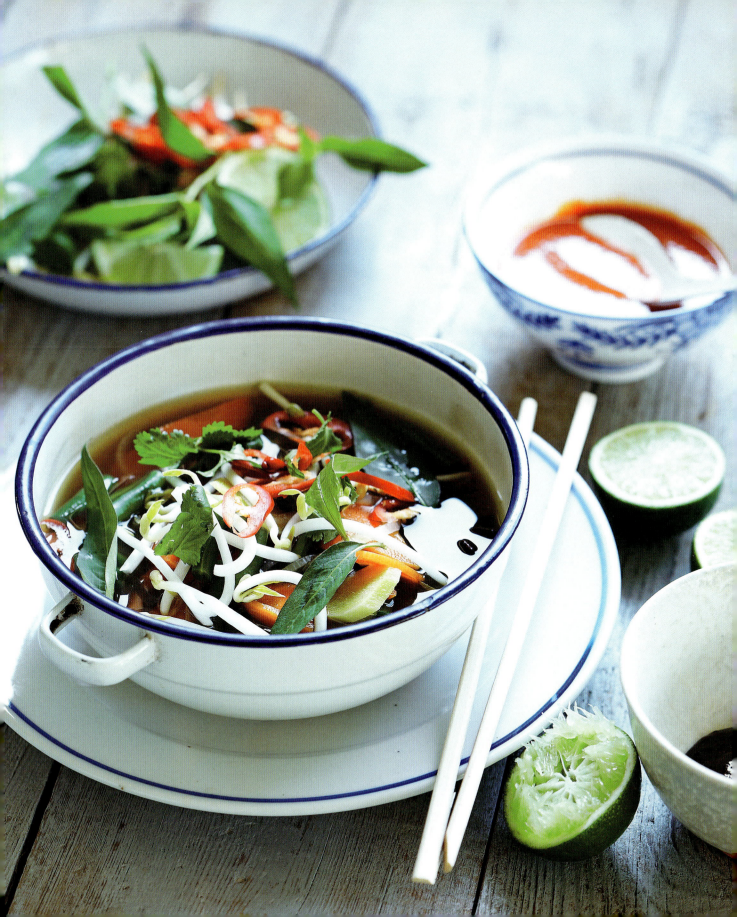

# SWEET
# THINGS

1 SERVE =
½ unit bread
½ unit dairy
1 unit fruit
2 units fats

cooking oil spray

1 bunch rhubarb, stalks trimmed and
   cut into 3 cm lengths

4 granny smith apples (about 600 g),
   peeled, cored and cut into 2 cm
   thick slices

3 tablespoons caster sugar or
   powdered sweetener

1 teaspoon ground ginger

1 teaspoon mixed spice

600 g reduced-fat vanilla yoghurt

CRUMBLE TOPPING

40 g hazelnuts

¾ cup (60 g) rolled oats

1 tablespoon plain flour

2 tablespoons honey, warmed

1½ tablespoons light
   margarine, melted

# Apple and rhubarb crumble with honey, oats and hazelnuts

SERVES 6  PREP **20 mins**  COOK **40 mins**

**The classic combination of apples and rhubarb, spiced with ginger, makes for a delicious crumble. You can cook this in individual 165 ml capacity ramekins or a 1 litre baking dish: the cooking time will be the same.**

1 Preheat the oven to 180°C and spray the dish/es with cooking oil.

2 For the crumble topping, roast the hazelnuts on a baking tray for 8–10 minutes until the skins loosen. Wrap the hazelnuts in a tea towel and rub off the skins. Roughly chop, then place in a bowl with the oats, flour, honey and margarine and mix well to combine.

3 Meanwhile, place a saucepan over low heat and add the rhubarb, apple, sugar or sweetener, ginger, mixed spice and 2 tablespoons water. Stir well, then cover and cook for 6–7 minutes until the fruit starts to soften. Remove the lid and continue to cook for a further 4–5 minutes until the fruit is tender but retains some shape. Spoon the mixture into the dish/es.

4 Sprinkle the crumble mixture over the fruit, place the dish/es on a baking tray and bake in the oven for 25–30 minutes until golden. Serve hot or warm with yoghurt.

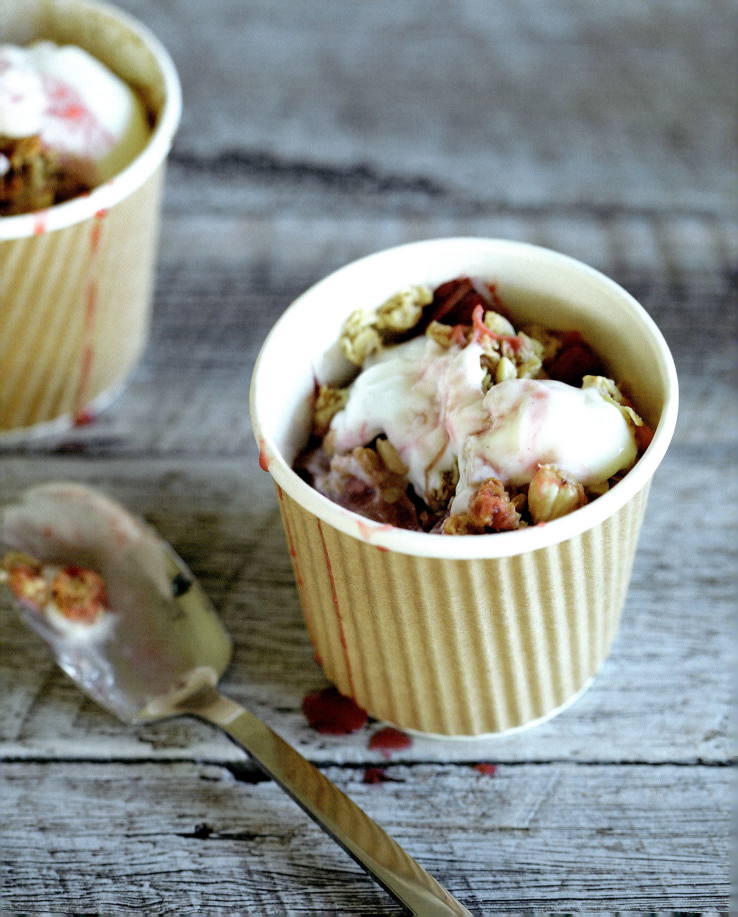

# Ricotta and sultana filo rolls with berry salsa

SERVES 4  PREP **20 mins**  COOK **25 mins**

1½ cups (300 g) fresh
  reduced-fat ricotta
¾ cup (150 g) reduced-fat
  cottage cheese
2 small eggs, lightly beaten
3 tablespoons sultanas, chopped
1 tablespoon honey
1 teaspoon vanilla extract or essence
½ teaspoon ground nutmeg
finely grated zest and juice
  of ½ lemon
6 sheets filo pastry
cooking oil spray
300 g fresh or frozen blueberries
  or blackberries
1½ tablespoons powdered sweetener
icing sugar, for dusting

**Inspired by a pancake dessert called a blintz, this low-carb version works perfectly well with filo pastry. Look for fresh filo in the chilled section of your supermarket as it's much easier to work with.**

1 Preheat the oven to 200°C and line a baking tray with baking paper.

2 Place the ricotta, cottage cheese, beaten egg, sultanas, honey, vanilla, nutmeg and lemon zest in a bowl and mix well to combine.

3 Lay a sheet of filo on a clean work surface and spray with cooking oil. Fold the sheet in half from the long end, and cut in half lengthways. Spoon a little of the cheese mixture along the short edge, leaving space at the ends so the filling does not spill out. Tuck in the ends, then roll up to enclose. Repeat with the remaining filo and cheese mixture to make twelve rolls. Place on the prepared tray, seam-side down, spray with cooking oil and bake for 20–25 minutes until the pastry is golden and crisp.

4 Meanwhile, for the salsa, place the berries, sweetener and lemon juice in a small saucepan and cook over medium heat for 5–6 minutes.

5 Serve three rolls per person, dusted lightly with icing sugar, with the warm berry salsa on top.

Tip: Try other spices such as ground cinnamon, cloves or cardamom for a different flavour.

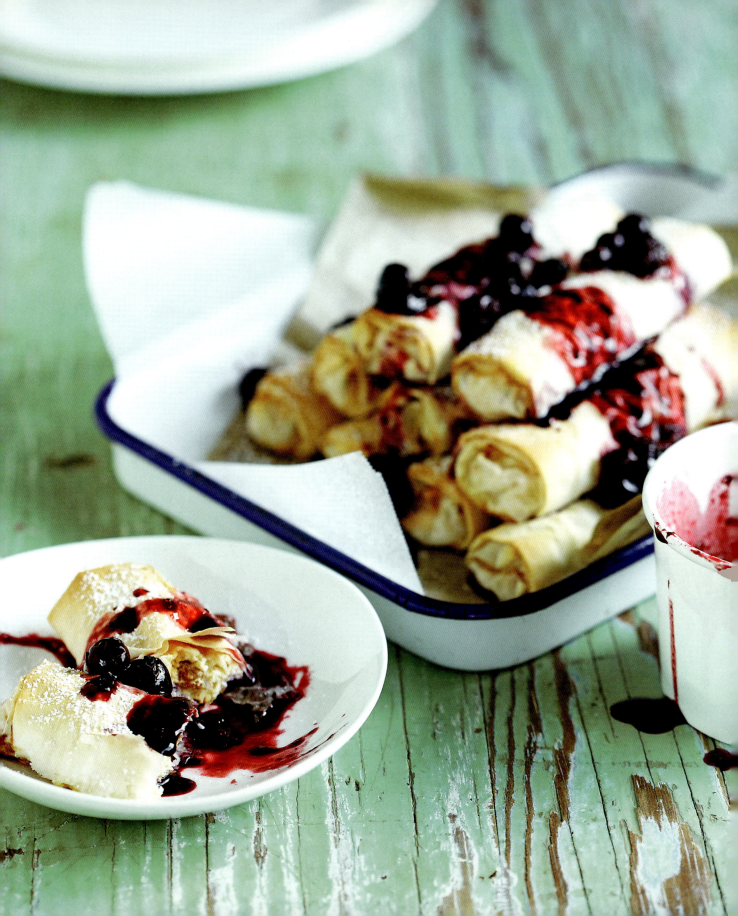

1 SERVE =
¼ unit dairy
½ unit fruit

# Mango and passionfruit frozen yoghurt pops

MAKES 8  PREP **10 mins**  FREEZE **6 hours**

2 cups (400 g) diced mango

2 cups (560 g) reduced-fat passionfruit yoghurt

3 tablespoons powdered sweetener

2 tablespoons lemon juice (optional)

**A great way to use in-season fruit, these yoghurt pops are a winner for young and old alike. Use any combination of fruit and yoghurt that you have on hand. They will keep for up to 2 weeks in the freezer.**

1 Place the mango in the bowl of a food processor and process until smooth. Add the yoghurt and sweetener and process until combined. Taste and add lemon juice if desired.

2 Pour into eight popsicle moulds and insert the sticks. Freeze for 6 hours or overnight.

**Tip:** If you don't have popsicle moulds, pour the mixture into small paper cups, cover with plastic wrap and poke an ice-cream stick through into the yoghurt. To eat, simply remove the plastic wrap and peel away the paper cup.

**Variations**

RASPBERRY AND CHOCOLATE: replace the mango with 2 cups (300 g) frozen raspberries, use reduced-fat chocolate yoghurt and omit the lemon juice.

BANANA AND HONEY: replace the mango with 2 cups (300 g) chopped ripe banana and use reduced-fat vanilla yoghurt. Add 2 tablespoons of honey instead of the sweetener, and omit the lemon juice if you like.

MIXED BERRY: replace the mango with 2 cups (300 g) frozen mixed berries and use reduced-fat strawberry yoghurt.

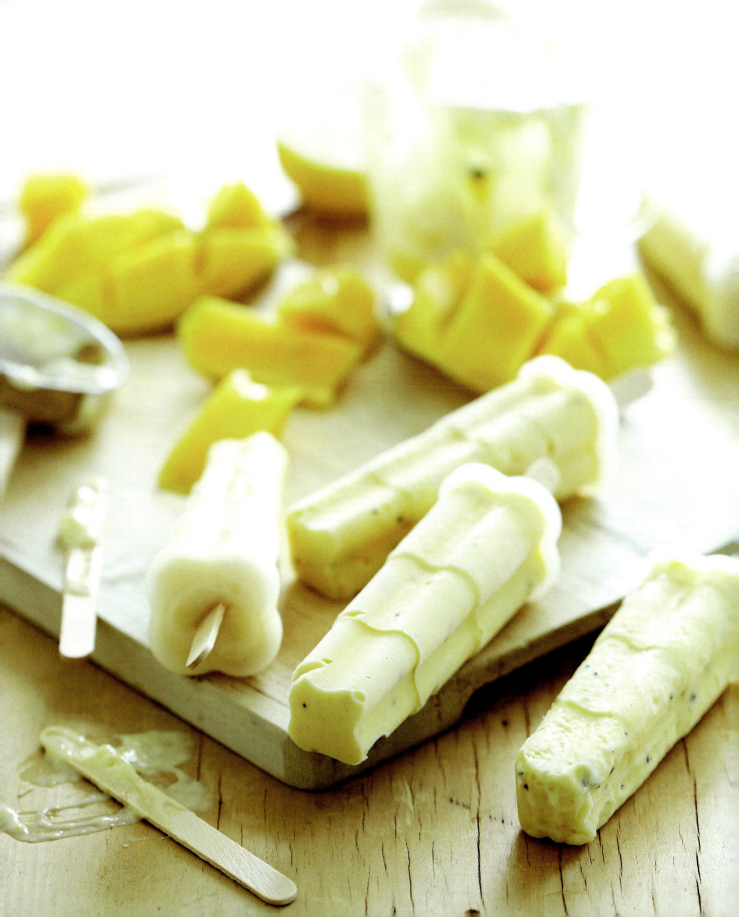

1 SERVE =
½ unit bread
½ unit dairy
1 unit fruit
1 unit fats

# Spiced pear and date strudel

SERVES 6  PREP **20 mins**  COOK **25 mins**

1 × 400 g tin pie pears with
   no added sugar
40 g chopped walnuts
3 tablespoons roughly chopped
   dried pitted dates
½ teaspoon ground cinnamon, plus
   extra for serving (optional)
½ teaspoon ground nutmeg
   or ground cloves
½ teaspoon ground ginger
1 tablespoon honey
6 sheets filo pastry
cooking oil spray
icing sugar, for dusting
600 g reduced-fat vanilla yoghurt

**A quick dessert to make if you're having friends over. Prepare the filling in advance, then roll the strudel and pop it in the oven to cook while you're eating your main meal.**

1 Preheat the oven to 180°C. Line a baking tray with baking paper.

2 Combine the pears, walnuts, dates, ground spices and honey in a medium-sized bowl.

3 On a clean work surface, stack the pastry sheets on top of one another, spraying cooking oil between each sheet. Spoon the pear mixture along the short edge, leaving a 5 cm border. Fold in the sides, then roll up tightly to enclose the filling. Place the roll, seam-side down, on the prepared tray.

4 Spray lightly with cooking oil, then bake for 20–25 minutes until the pastry is golden and crisp. Dust lightly with icing sugar, then cut into slices. Serve warm with yoghurt and sprinkled with extra cinnamon, if liked.

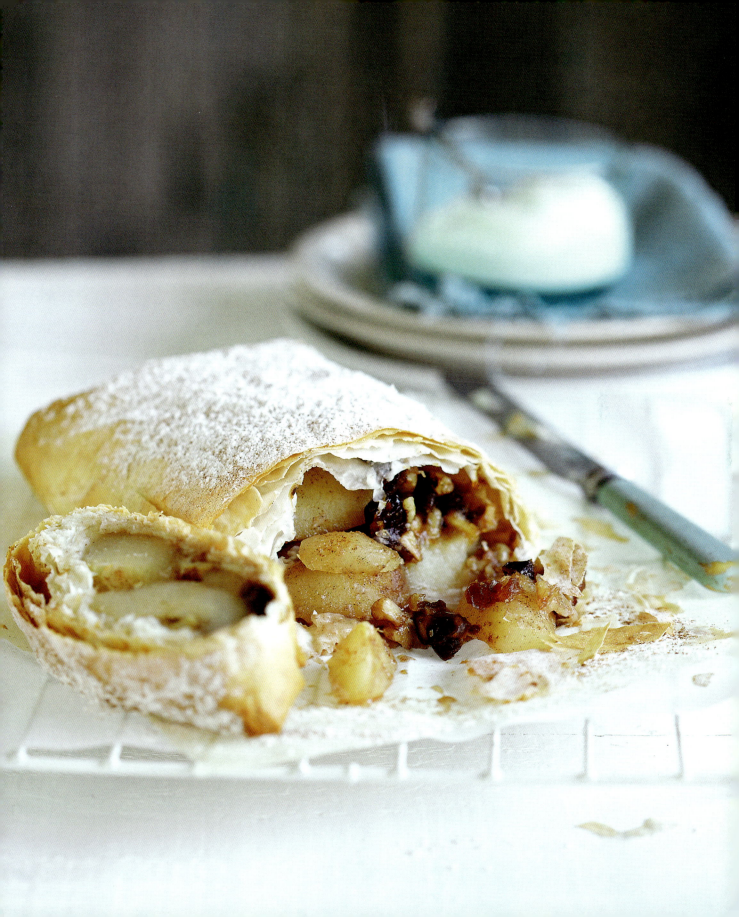

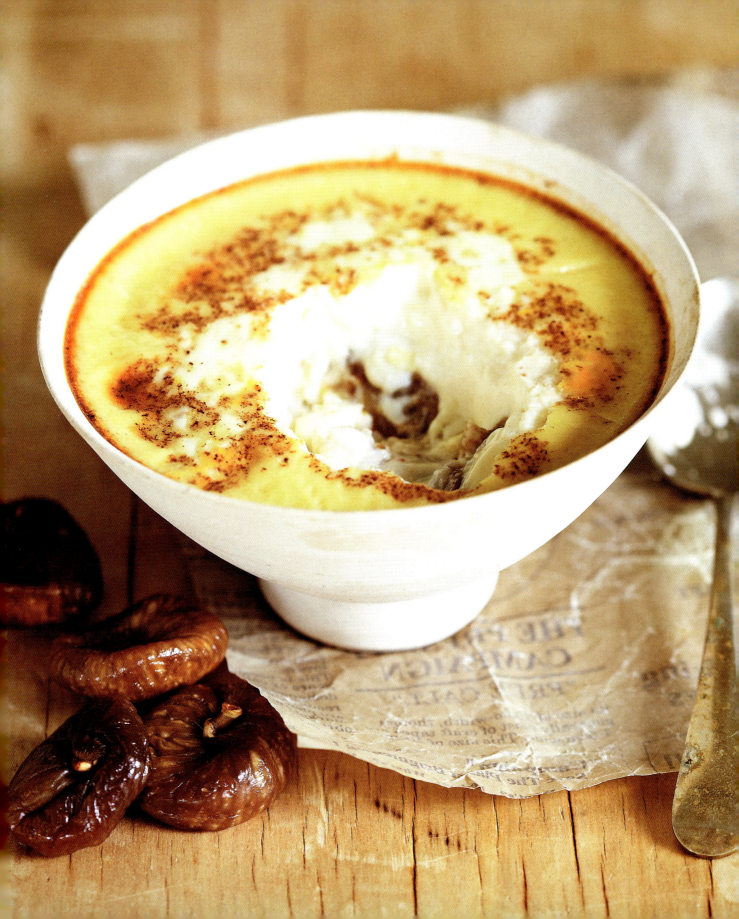

**1 SERVE =**
¼ unit protein
¼ unit bread
¼ unit dairy
½ unit fruit

cooking oil spray
⅔ cup (125 g) cooked white rice
60 g chopped dried figs
3 eggs
4 tablespoons caster sugar or
    powdered sweetener
½ teaspoon ground ginger
1 teaspoon vanilla extract or essence
2 cups (500 ml) reduced-fat milk
¼ teaspoon ground nutmeg

# Rice puddings with ginger and figs

SERVES 6  PREP **10 mins**  COOK **50 mins, plus cooling time**

**You'll need six ½ cup (125 ml) capacity ramekins for this comforting dessert. Allow it to rest for 15 minutes before eating, as the custard will continue to set as it cools.**

1 Preheat the oven to 180°C and spray the ramekins with cooking oil.

2 Divide the rice and chopped fig among the ramekins and place them in a deep roasting tin. Whisk the eggs with the sugar or sweetener, ginger and vanilla until combined, then gently stir in the milk. Divide the milk mixture among the ramekins.

3 Pour enough hot water into the roasting tin to come halfway up the sides of the ramekins. Place the tin in the oven and cook for 15 minutes, then gently stir each custard with a fork to evenly distribute the rice and fruit. Cook for another 15 minutes and stir the custards again. Cook for a further 15–20 minutes until the puddings are just set and a knife inserted into the centre comes out clean. Allow to cool for 15 minutes before serving dusted with nutmeg. They can also be served chilled.

Tip: Replace the figs with 60 g sultanas if you prefer.

# Ginger and fig loaf

MAKES 14 SLICES  PREP **15 mins**  COOK **50 mins**

½ cup (125 ml) reduced-fat milk
**40 g light margarine**
**4 tablespoons brown sugar
  or powdered sweetener**
**½ cup (100 g) dried figs, chopped**
**1 egg**
**1¼ cups (185 g) self-raising
  flour, sifted**
**2 teaspoons ground ginger**
**1 teaspoon ground cinnamon**

**This simple spiced fruit loaf is as good as you'll get at your local cafe at a fraction of the price, and is delicious served as is or lightly toasted. Wrap slices individually in plastic wrap and freeze for up to 2 weeks.**

1 Preheat the oven to 160°C. Line a 21 cm × 9 cm loaf tin with baking paper, extending 5 cm above the rim on the long sides to use as handles.

2 Place the milk and margarine in a saucepan over medium heat. When the margarine has melted, pour the mixture into a heatproof bowl. Stir in the sugar or sweetener and fig, mixing until the sugar dissolves. Whisk in the egg, then add the flour and ground spices, stirring until just combined.

3 Spoon the mixture into the prepared tin and level the top, then bake for 45–50 minutes until a skewer inserted in the centre comes out clean. Leave to cool in the tin for 15 minutes, then turn out onto a rack and allow to cool completely. Slice and serve.

**Tip:** Try this with other dried fruits, such as dates or sultanas.

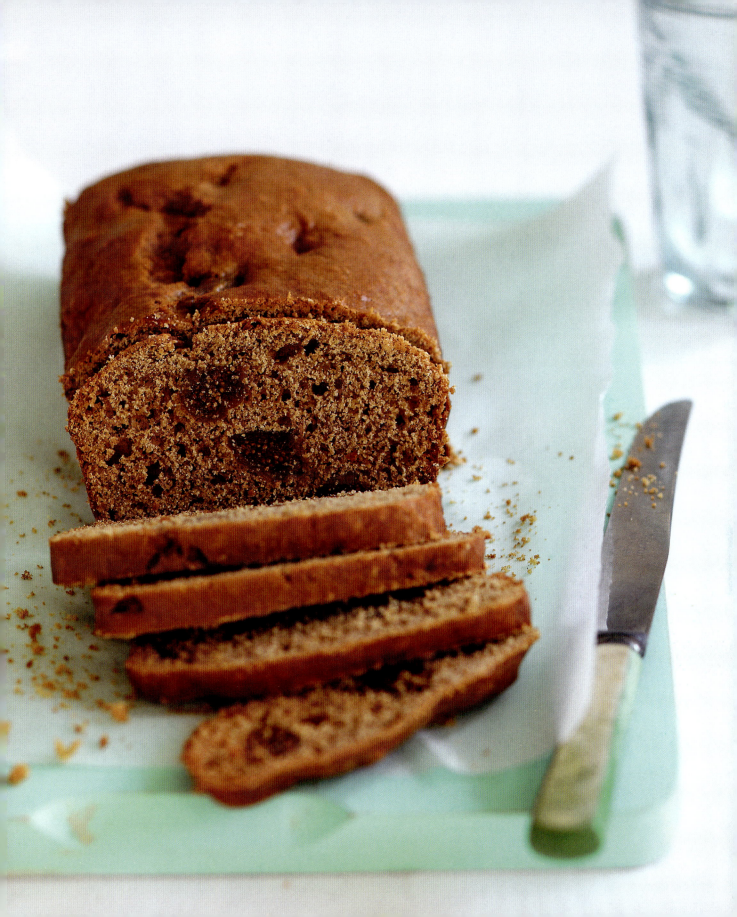

**1 SERVE =**
¼ unit protein
1 unit dairy
½ unit fruit
½ unit fats

1 tablespoon flaked almonds
3 cups (600 g) fresh
    reduced-fat ricotta
2½ tablespoons powdered sweetener
2 eggs
2 teaspoons ground ginger
½ teaspoon ground cardamom
1½ teaspoons vanilla extract
    or essence
1 tablespoon honey
1 × 390 g tin apricot halves in fruit
    juice, drained, juice reserved

# Baked spiced ricotta with apricots

SERVES 4  PREP **10 mins**  COOK **1 hour 10 mins, plus cooling time**

**Being low in fat, ricotta is an excellent option for dessert. Use a high-sided bread tin for this recipe, as the mixture rises during cooking and then settles as it cools. Allow the ricotta to cool to room temperature before eating as the texture and flavour will improve.**

1 Preheat oven to 180°C and line a 15 cm × 8.5 cm high-sided bread tin with baking paper extending over the sides.

2 Roast the flaked almonds on a baking tray for 5–6 minutes until lightly golden, then set aside.

3 Place the ricotta, powdered sweetener, eggs, ginger, cardamom, and vanilla in the bowl of a food processor and mix until smooth. Alternatively, beat the ingredients with hand-held electric beaters until smooth.

4 Spoon the mixture into the prepared tin and smooth the top. Bake for 55–60 minutes until puffed and golden and a skewer inserted into the centre comes out clean.

5 Remove from the oven and allow to cool in the tin for 20 minutes. Gently lift the baked ricotta from the tin using the overhanging baking paper, then set aside to cool to room temperature or refrigerate until ready to use.

6 Place the honey and 2 tablespoons of the reserved apricot juice in a bowl and stir to combine.

7 Cut the ricotta into four squares and divide among plates. Top each square with four apricot halves, then drizzle over some honey syrup and scatter over the almonds.

**Tip:** Try adding a teaspoon of rosewater to the syrup, and garnish with some chopped roast pistachios instead of the almonds.

1 cup (150 g) plain flour
4 tablespoons powdered sweetener
3 tablespoons polenta
½ teaspoon baking powder
finely grated zest of 2 lemons
1 teaspoon mixed spice
2 teaspoons poppy seeds
2 small eggs
1 tablespoon canola oil

# Lemon and poppy-seed biscotti

MAKES 24  PREP **30 mins, plus cooling time**  COOK **50 mins**

**A great accompaniment to an afternoon cup of tea, these biscotti are made for dunking. Store in an airtight container for up to 3 days, or freeze in batches for up to 2 weeks.**

1 Preheat the oven to 160°C and line a baking tray with baking paper.

2 Combine the flour, sweetener, polenta, baking powder, lemon zest, mixed spice and poppy seeds in a large bowl. Whisk the eggs and oil together, then add to the flour mixture and stir until a soft dough forms.

3 Turn out the dough onto a floured work surface and gently knead to bring it together. Shape into a 30 cm × 3 cm log and place on the prepared tray.

4 Bake for 20–25 minutes until the log is almost firm when pressed on top. Remove from the oven and allow to cool on the tray for 15 minutes. Reduce the oven temperature to 150°C.

5 Transfer the log to a chopping board and cut on the diagonal into 1.5 cm thick slices. Place the biscotti pieces, standing upright, on the baking tray. Return to the oven and bake for a further 20–25 minutes until lightly coloured and dry, then transfer to a wire rack to cool.

Tip: For a different flavour combination, replace the mixed spice with the same amount of cinnamon, the lemon zest with 1 teaspoon vanilla extract or essence and omit the poppy seeds.

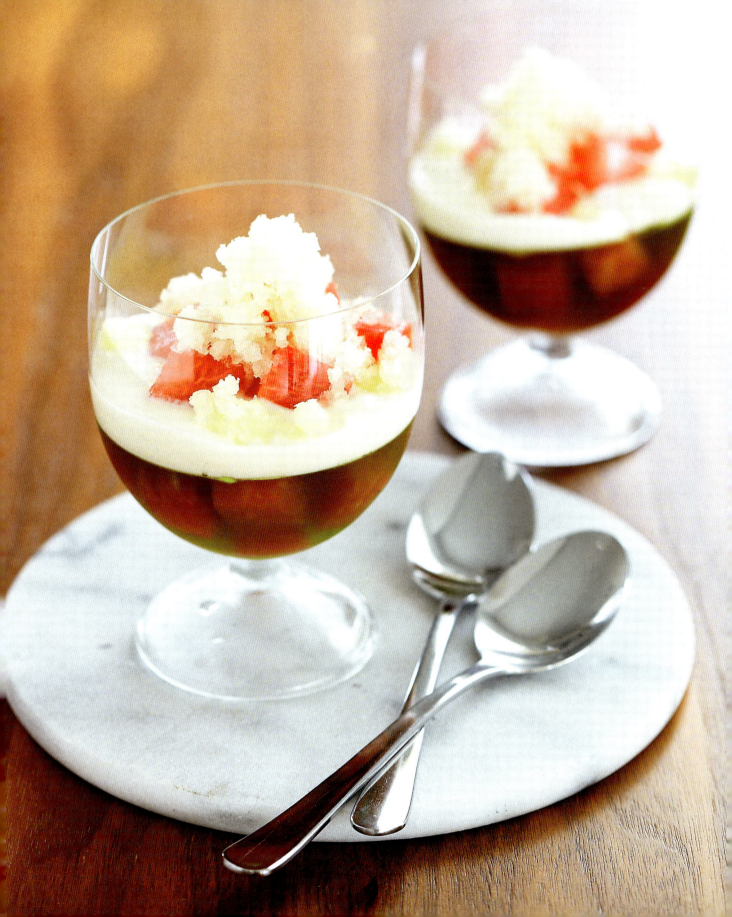

3 tablespoons caster sugar
finely grated zest and juice of 2 limes
juice of 3 lemons, approximately
6 g low-joule apple or
   lime jelly crystals
1 cup (250 ml) boiling water
450 g watermelon, seeded and
   cut into 2 cm dice
250 g reduced-fat vanilla yoghurt

# Apple and watermelon jelly with lemon-lime granita

SERVES 6  PREP **10 mins, plus refrigerating and freezing time**
COOK **5 mins**

**Creamy, refreshing and light, this dessert makes an impressive finish to a meal.**

1 Place the sugar, lime zest and ½ cup (125 ml) water in a small saucepan and stir over low heat until the sugar dissolves. Bring to the boil, then reduce the heat and simmer for 5 minutes. Remove from the heat and strain into a bowl, discarding the zest. Refrigerate the sugar syrup for 30 minutes.

2 Combine the lime juice with enough lemon juice to make up 200 ml, and mix well into the sugar syrup. Pour the mixture into a shallow container and freeze for 45 minutes. Stir with a fork, then return to the freezer for 35–40 minutes, then stir again. Continue this process for 2–3 hours until the granita is frozen.

3 Meanwhile, place the jelly crystals and the boiling water into a bowl and stir until dissolved. Add 1 cup (250 ml) cold water and stir to combine. Divide half the watermelon among six large glasses and pour over the jelly. Chill for 2–3 hours until set.

4 To serve, spoon 2 tablespoons of the yoghurt over each glass of jelly, then top with the remaining watermelon and 2 tablespoons of lemon-lime granita.

**Tip:** The leftover granita will keep in the freezer for 3 days. Use it to make lemonade or to flavour iced tea.

2 egg whites, at room temperature
½ cup (110 g) caster sugar
1 mango, peeled and stone removed,
    thinly sliced
600 g reduced-fat
    passionfruit yoghurt
4 passionfruit, pulp removed

# Eton mess with passionfruit and mango

**SERVES 6** PREP **15 mins** COOK **1 hour, plus cooling time**

**As its name suggests, this dessert, made with chunks of meringue mixed with yoghurt and fresh fruit, is a little messy. The meringue will keep for a few days in an airtight container, making for a quick fix in a dessert emergency.**

1 Preheat the oven to 150°C and line a baking tray with baking paper.

2 Beat the eggwhites and a pinch of salt with hand-held electric beaters until soft peaks form. Add the sugar, a tablespoon at a time, beating well between each addition, until thick and glossy. Spoon the meringue mixture into six 8 cm mounds on the prepared tray. Place in the oven, then immediately reduce the temperature to 120°C and bake for 1 hour until crisp. Turn the oven off and leave the meringues in the oven to cool completely.

3 To serve, break the meringues into large pieces. Reserving a few slices of mango for garnish, layer the meringue, yoghurt, passionfruit and mango into large glasses, then top with the reserved mango.

**Tip:** Serve this with any in-season fruit: fresh berries and kiwifruit work particularly well.

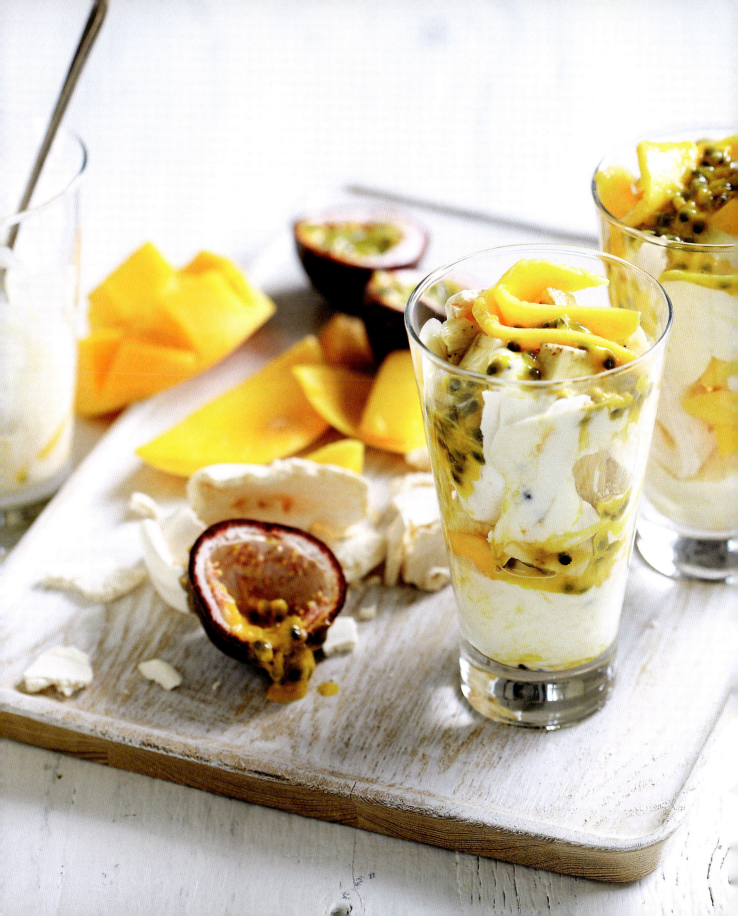

# Apple and cinnamon mini muffins

MAKES 24  PREP **10 mins**  COOK **17 mins**

cooking oil spray
3½ tablespoons powdered sweetener
3 teaspoons ground cinnamon
⅔ cup (100 g) wholemeal flour
⅔ cup (100 g) plain flour
3 teaspoons baking powder
2 eggs, lightly beaten
½ cup (125 ml) reduced-fat milk
   or reduced-fat buttermilk
1 small green apple, coarsely grated

**Delicately spiced, with just the right amount of sweetness, these muffins are the perfect mid-morning snack. Make a double batch and freeze some for later – they'll keep for up to 2 weeks.**

1 Preheat the oven to 180°C. Spray a 24-hole mini muffin pan with cooking oil.

2 Mix together the sweetener and cinnamon, then set aside 2 teaspoons of this mixture in a small bowl.

3 Combine the flours, baking powder and the remaining sugar and cinnamon in a large bowl. In another bowl, whisk the eggs and milk or buttermilk together, then add to the flour mixture along with the grated apple, and mix gently until just combined.

4 Spoon the batter into the muffin holes and sprinkle over the reserved cinnamon sugar. Bake for 15–17 minutes until golden and springy to the touch. Leave to cool in the tin for 5 minutes, then transfer to a wire rack to cool.

**Tip:** Try this version for something a little different: replace the grated apple with pear, and replace the cinnamon with ground ginger and mix with 2½ tablespoons shredded coconut and the sweetener. Reserve 2 teaspoons of this coconut mixture to use as a topping and add the rest in with the flour as above.

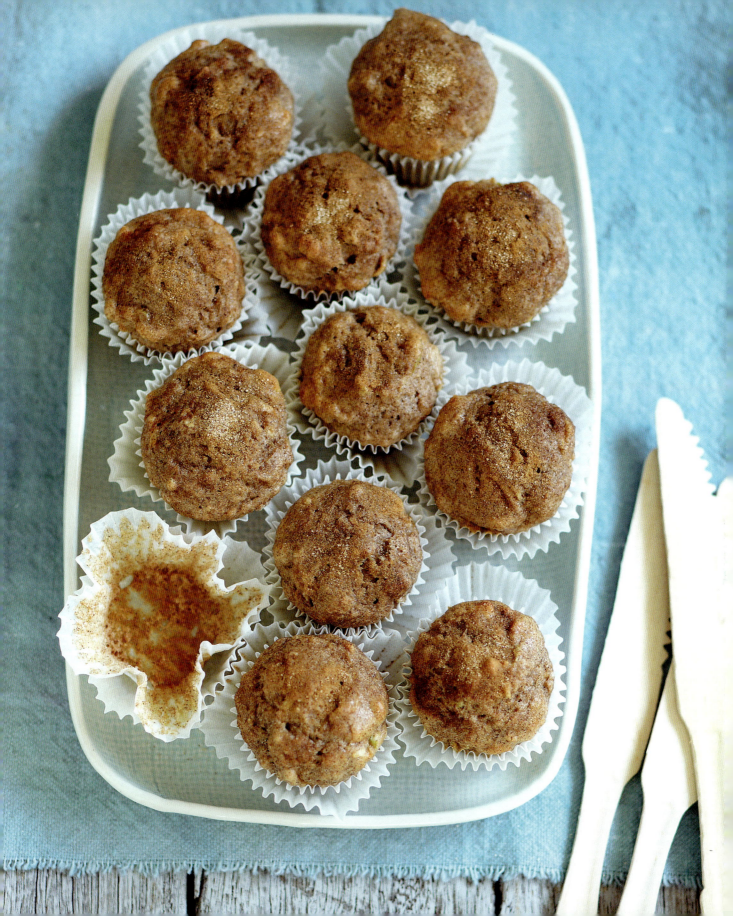

1 SERVE =
¼ unit protein
½ unit dairy
½ unit fruit

# Cinnamon and clove-spiced cherry custards

SERVES 4  PREP **10 mins**  COOK **50 mins**

1¼ cups (250 g) drained pitted
   black cherries in light syrup
2 cups (500 ml) reduced-fat milk
3 eggs
3 tablespoons caster sugar
1 teaspoon vanilla extract or essence
½ teaspoon ground cinnamon
large pinch ground cloves
icing sugar, for dusting

**A lovely dessert to serve when guests come around. You can buy pitted black cherries in tins from the supermarket.**

1 Preheat the oven to 160°C. Divide the cherries among four 165 ml ramekins or glasses.

2 Heat the milk in a saucepan until almost boiling, then remove from the heat and set aside.

3 In a large bowl, gently whisk the eggs, sugar, vanilla and spices until well combined but not frothy. Whisking constantly, pour the hot milk over the egg mixture in a slow steady stream and whisk gently until combined. Strain the mixture through a sieve into a bowl, then divide among the four ramekins. Using a spoon, skim away any bubbles from the surface.

4 Place the ramekins in a deep roasting tin, and pour enough hot water into the tin to come halfway up the sides of the ramekins. Bake for 35–45 minutes until the custard is just set with a slight wobble in the centre. Remove the ramekins from the tin and allow to cool.

5 Served chilled or at room temperature, lightly dusted with icing sugar.

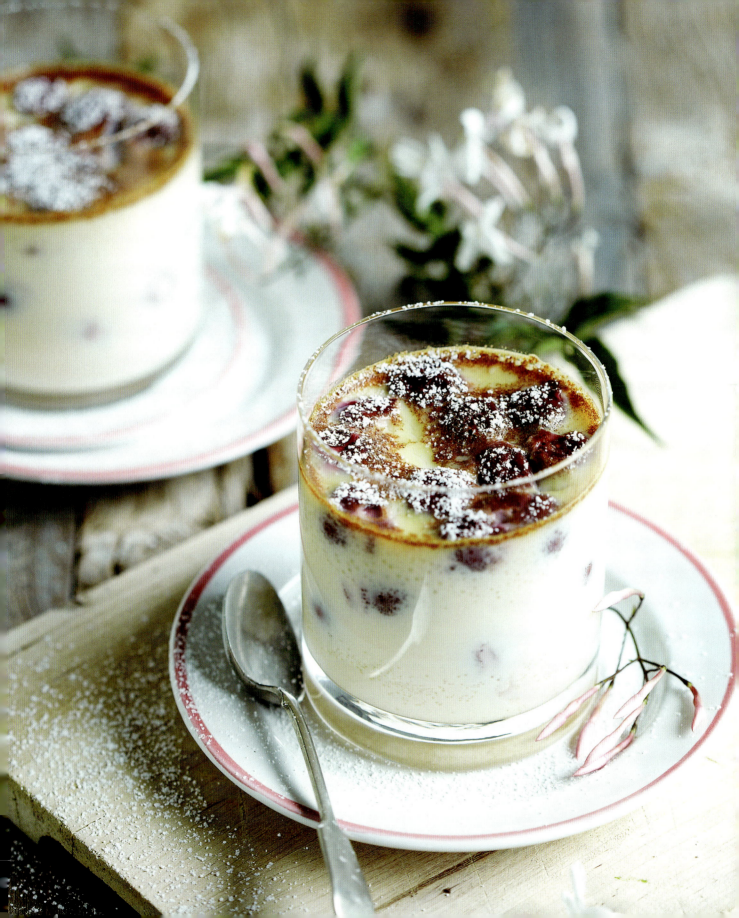

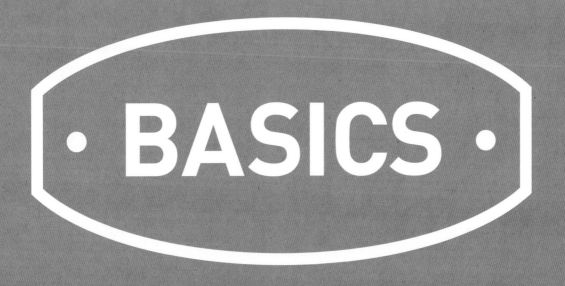

1 SERVE (80 G) =
¼ unit bread
1 unit vegetables
1½ units fats

40 g hazelnuts or almonds
3 red capsicums (peppers), trimmed,
   seeded and quartered
8 cloves garlic, unpeeled
2 tomatoes
1 slice stale bread, crusts removed,
   bread toasted
½–1 teaspoon sweet paprika
pinch cayenne pepper
1 tablespoon extra virgin olive oil
2–3 tablespoons red wine vinegar
   or sherry vinegar
basil leaves (optional), to serve

# Romesco sauce

MAKES 2 CUPS (540 G)  PREP **20 mins, plus standing time**  COOK **20 mins**

**This is a delicious roast capsicum sauce originating from Spain. It is commonly used to accompany seafood, but it goes just as well with chicken or pork or as a spread for sandwiches. It will keep refrigerated for 3–4 days.**

1 Preheat the oven to 180°C. Spread the nuts on a baking tray and roast for 8–10 minutes until golden. If using hazelnuts, wrap them in a tea towel and rub off the skins. Chop and set aside.

2 Preheat the oven grill to high.

3 Place the capsicum, skin-side up, under the grill in a single layer and cook for 8–10 minutes until the skin blackens and blisters. Transfer to a bowl, cover with plastic wrap and leave for 10 minutes to steam, then peel away the skin and discard, setting the flesh aside.

4 Meanwhile, reduce the oven grill to medium. Place the whole garlic cloves and tomatoes under the grill and cook, turning, for 6–8 minutes until blackened. Remove from the grill and, when cool enough to handle, peel off and discard the skins from the garlic and tomatoes. Seed the tomatoes and roughly chop.

5 Place the nuts in a blender or food processor and chop until finely ground. Add the garlic and tomato, bread, spices and olive oil and process until smooth. Season with salt and pepper, then add vinegar to taste. Serve with basil leaves mixed through, if liked.

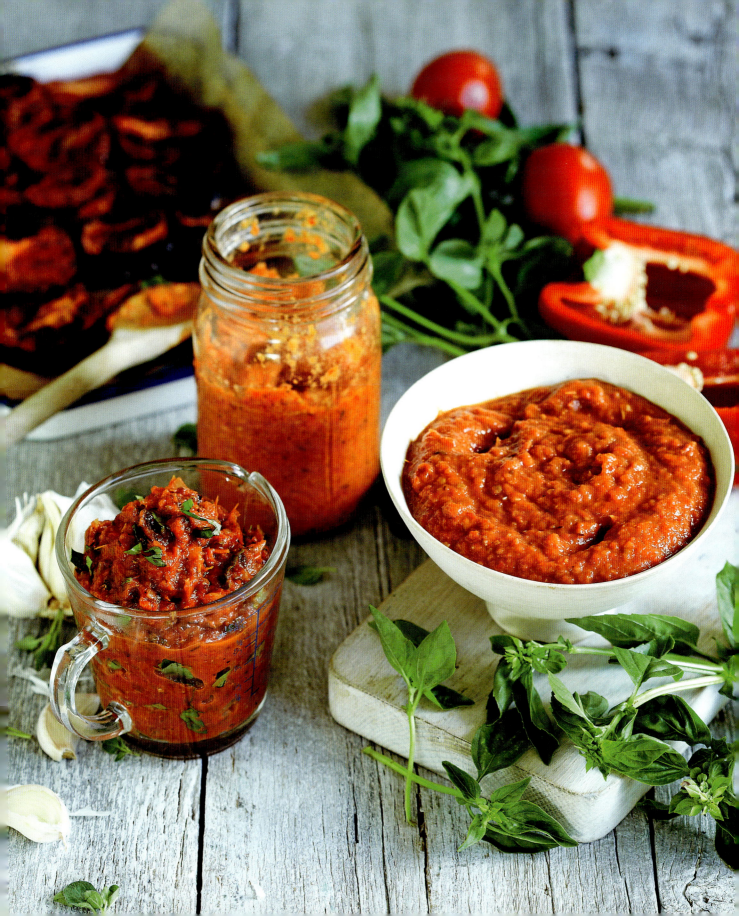

# Slow-roasted tomato sauce

**MAKES 2½ CUPS (625 ML)** PREP **15 mins**
COOK **1 hour 15 mins**

**This simple sauce is a great base that can be flavoured to suit any dish, especially pasta dishes (see right). Slow-roasting the tomatoes draws out their moisture and intensifies the flavour. Store the sauce in an airtight container in the fridge for 1 week, or in the freezer for 1 month.**

**1 kg ripe roma (plum) tomatoes, halved lengthways**
**4 cloves garlic, sliced**
**2 teaspoons brown sugar**
**cooking oil spray**
**1½ tablespoons red wine vinegar**

1 Preheat the oven to 170°C.

2 Place the tomatoes, cut-side up, in a roasting tin just large enough to hold them in a single layer. Scatter over the garlic and sugar, spray with cooking oil, then season to taste with salt and pepper and drizzle over the vinegar. Roast for 1 hour 15 minutes until soft and pulpy.

3 Remove from the oven and puree with a hand-held blender until smooth. Taste and adjust the seasonings, then set aside to cool before storing.

## Variations

TO MAKE BASIL AND OLIVE PASTA SAUCE:
Fry 1 small, finely chopped onion with 1 tablespoon olive oil and 2 teaspoons dried oregano over medium heat for 7–8 minutes until the onion is very soft. Add 1 quantity slow-roasted tomato sauce and 3 tablespoons chopped black olives and simmer for 5 minutes. Stir through a handful of chopped basil just before serving.

**1 serve = ½ unit vegetables, 1 unit fats**

TO MAKE ANCHOVY AND PARSLEY PASTA SAUCE:
Fry 1 small, finely chopped onion with 1 tablespoon olive oil and 4 drained and chopped anchovy fillets over medium heat for 7–8 minutes until the onion is very soft. Add 1 quantity slow-roasted tomato sauce, a small handful chopped flat-leaf parsley and the finely grated zest of 1 lemon and simmer for 5 minutes.

**1 serve = 2 units vegetables, 1½ units fats**

TO MAKE CHILLI AND CAPER PASTA SAUCE:
Fry 1 small, finely chopped onion with 1 tablespoon olive oil, 1 tablespoon chopped rosemary and ½ teaspoon dried chilli flakes over medium heat for 7–8 minutes until the onion is very soft. Add 1 quantity slow-roasted tomato sauce and 3 tablespoons drained and chopped capers and simmer for 5 minutes.

**1 serve = ½ unit vegetables, 1 unit fats**

TO MAKE SAUCE FOR A PIZZA BASE:
Combine 1 cup (250 ml) slow-roasted tomato sauce with 2 tablespoons salt-reduced tomato paste (puree) and 1 tablespoon dried Italian herbs and mix well.

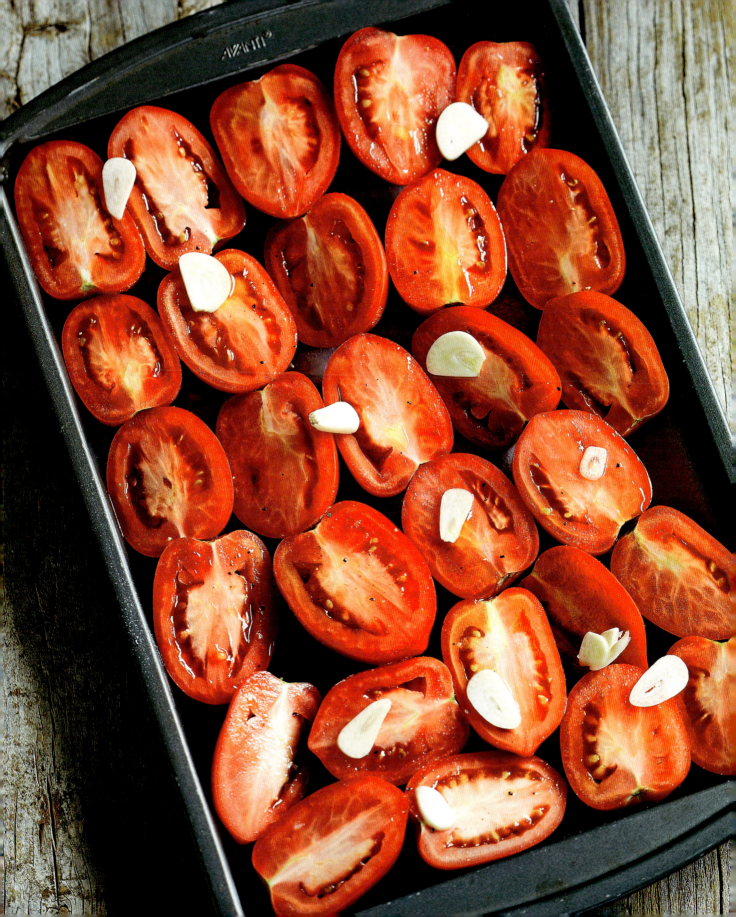

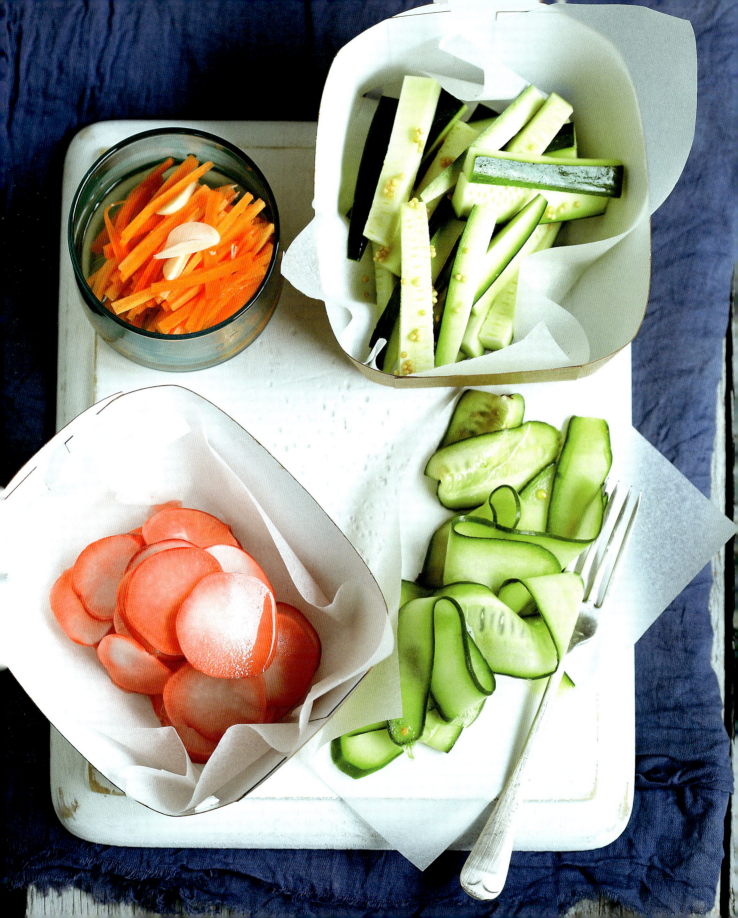

These delicious and versatile pickles can be used in sandwiches, salads or stir-fries to add a fresh, crunchy, sweet–sour note. You only need a small amount to add a punch of flavour, so these are a great 'free-list' food. They will keep refrigerated for up to 2 weeks.

PREP **10 mins**  COOK **5 mins, plus cooling time**

# Pickled carrot

### MAKES 350 G

**435 ml rice vinegar or white vinegar**
**1 tablespoon caster sugar or powdered sweetener**
**1 teaspoon salt**
**350 g carrots, cut into 2 mm thick matchsticks**
**3 cloves garlic, thinly sliced**

1 Bring the vinegar, sugar or sweetener, salt and 165 ml water to the boil in a saucepan, then reduce the heat and simmer for 5 minutes. Remove from the heat and set aside to cool.

2 Place the carrot and garlic slices into an airtight container or jar. Pour over the cooled liquid and seal tightly. For the best flavour, allow to stand for 1 day before eating.

# Pickled radish

### MAKES 3 CUPS (600 G)

**1½ cups (375 ml) rice vinegar or white vinegar**
**1 tablespoon caster sugar or powdered sweetener**
**1 teaspoon salt**
**2 bunches (600 g) radishes, trimmed and**
   **cut into thin rounds**
**2 teaspoons finely sliced ginger**
**pinch dried chilli flakes (optional)**

1 Bring the vinegar, sugar or sweetener, salt and 165 ml water to the boil in a saucepan, then reduce the heat and simmer for 5 minutes. Remove from the heat and set aside to cool.

2 Place the radish, ginger and chilli flakes (if using) into an airtight container or jar. Pour over the cooled liquid and seal tightly. For the best flavour, allow to stand for 1 day before eating.

# Pickled zucchini

### MAKES 400 G

**1½ cups (375 ml) rice vinegar or white vinegar**
**1 tablespoon caster sugar or powdered sweetener**
**1 teaspoon salt**
**400 g zucchinis (courgettes), cut into batons**
**1 teaspoon yellow mustard seeds**

1 Bring the vinegar, sugar or sweetener, salt and 165 ml water to the boil in a saucepan, then reduce the heat and simmer for 5 minutes. Remove from the heat and set aside to cool.

2 Place the zucchini and mustard seeds into an airtight container or jar. Pour over the cooled liquid and seal tightly. For the best flavour, allow to stand for 1 day before eating.

# Pickled cucumber

### MAKES 500 G

**1½ cups (375 ml) rice vinegar or white vinegar**
**1 tablespoon caster sugar or powdered sweetener**
**1 teaspoon salt**
**3–4 (500 g) Lebanese (small) cucumbers, cut into**
   **wide ribbons with a vegetable peeler**
**pinch dried chilli flakes**

1 Bring the vinegar, sugar or sweetener, salt and 165 ml water to the boil in a saucepan, then reduce the heat and simmer for 5 minutes. Remove from the heat and set aside to cool.

2 Place the cucumber and chilli flakes into an airtight container or jar. Pour over the cooled liquid and seal tightly. For the best flavour, allow to stand for 1 day before eating.

# Spiced eggplant dip

MAKES 520 G  PREP **10 mins, plus cooling time**
COOK **10 mins**

**Similar to baba ghanoush, this spicy eggplant dip is smoky and fresh. Eat with warmed pita bread or serve alongside Indian or Middle Eastern dishes. It will keep for up to 3 days in the fridge.**

2 eggplants (aubergines)
1–2 tomatoes, seeded and chopped
2 spring onions, trimmed and finely sliced
½ teaspoon Garam Masala (see page 208)
2–3 teaspoons lemon juice
pinch cayenne pepper or chilli powder

1 Roast the eggplants over a flame, turning often, for 10 minutes until blackened. Alternatively, roast the eggplants in a preheated 200°C oven for 30 minutes until soft. Allow to cool, then peel away the skin.

2 Roughly chop the flesh, or puree in a food processor, then add the remaining ingredients and combine. Season to taste with salt and pepper.

**Tip:** Try adding different spices such as ground cumin or coriander, or a clove of crushed garlic. Fresh herbs such as coriander or mint stirred through would work well too.

# Carrot dip

MAKES APPROX 500 G  PREP **10 mins**  COOK **10 mins**

**Gently spiced with a hint of sweetness, this dip also works well as a spread for sandwiches and has very few calories. Try it anywhere you would normally use mayo, avocado or butter. It will keep for up to 2 days in the fridge.**

500 g carrots, chopped
3 teaspoons honey
3–4 teaspoons lemon juice
½ teaspoon ground cumin
½ teaspoon sweet paprika

1 Bring a large saucepan of water to the boil and add the carrot. Cook for 6–7 minutes until the carrot is soft but not falling apart, then drain well.

2 Place the carrot and the remaining ingredients in a blender and season with salt and pepper. Blend until smooth, then adjust the seasonings to taste by adding more lemon juice or spices, if desired.

**Tip:** Try adding different spices, such as ground chilli or cinnamon, or add a tablespoon of chopped fresh mint or parsley or a tablespoon of reduced-fat plain yoghurt.

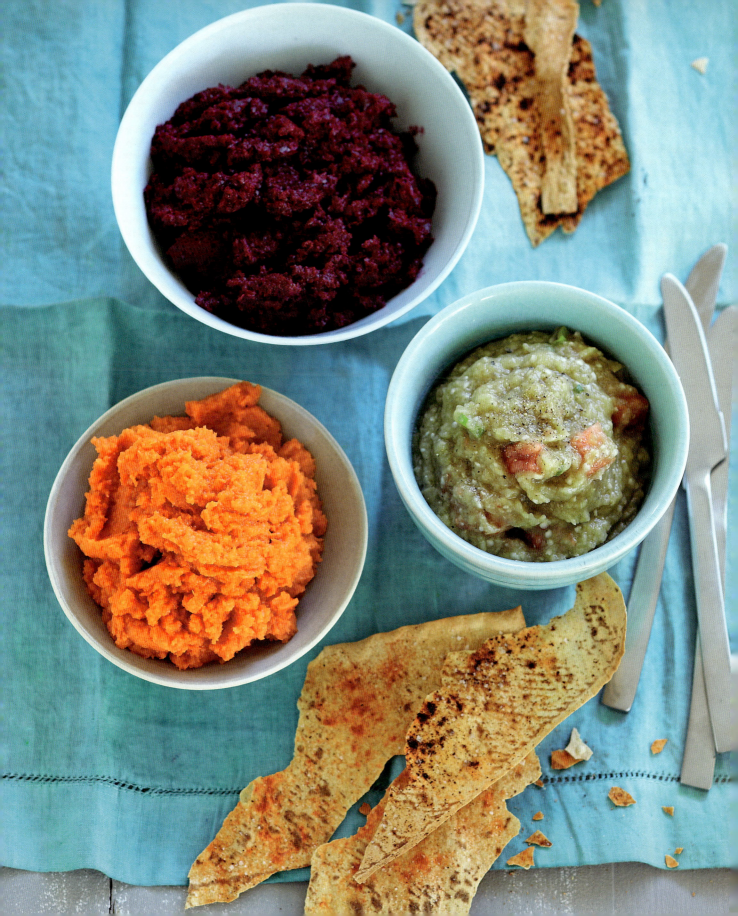

# Roast beetroot dip

(pictured on previous page)

MAKES 2 CUPS (400 G)  PREP **15 mins**  COOK **1 hour**

Vibrant and silky, this dip is extremely versatile – you can spread it on sandwiches, serve it with red meat or just eat it with a spoon. It will keep for up to 3 days in the fridge.

1 bunch (600 g) large beetroot, trimmed and scrubbed
5 cloves garlic, unpeeled
3 tablespoons reduced-fat Greek-style yoghurt
1–2 teaspoons red wine vinegar
1 tablespoon chopped mint or 2 teaspoons dried mint

1 Preheat the oven to 200°C.

2 Wrap the beetroot and garlic in separate foil parcels and place on a baking tray. Roast for 40 minutes, then remove the garlic and continue to roast the beetroot for a further 15–20 minutes until tender when pierced with a skewer.

3 When cool enough to handle, peel off the beetroot skin and roughly chop the flesh. Squeeze the garlic from their skins and add to the bowl of a food processor, along with the beetroot.

4 Process to a rough consistency, then add the yoghurt, vinegar and mint and season to taste with salt and pepper. Pulse a few times to combine, then adjust the seasonings to taste by adding more vinegar or mint, if desired.

# Zucchini hummus

MAKES 320 G  PREP **15 mins**

Zucchini hummus is incredibly tasty, with far less fat than the chickpea version. Squeeze out as much moisture from the zucchini as you can, as this will affect the flavour balance. Adjust spices and seasonings to taste.

2 medium-sized zucchinis (courgettes), coarsely grated
1 tablespoon tahini
1 tablespoon lemon juice
2 teaspoons extra virgin olive oil
1 clove garlic, very finely chopped
½ teaspoon ground cumin
pinch cayenne pepper or chilli powder

1 Squeeze out as much liquid as possible from the grated zucchini, then combine all the ingredients in the bowl of a food processor and mix until smooth, stopping a few times to scrape down the side of the bowl. Season to taste with salt and pepper, then adjust the seasonings to taste by adding more tahini, lemon juice or spices, if desired.

# Thai green curry paste

**MAKES ENOUGH FOR A CURRY FOR 4 PEOPLE**
PREP **15 mins** COOK **10 mins**

Making your own curry paste is not only better for you, as there are no oil or preservatives added, but the flavour is unrivalled. Shrimp paste (belacan) is available from Asian food stores. This curry paste will keep in the freezer for up to 1 month.

1 teaspoon shrimp paste (belacan), optional
2–3 tablespoons chopped small green chilli
2 tablespoons chopped lemongrass
3 tablespoons chopped red shallots
   or red (Spanish) onion
2 tablespoons chopped garlic
1 tablespoon grated ginger
1 tablespoon chopped coriander roots and stems
1 teaspoon ground coriander
½ teaspoon ground cumin
½ teaspoon ground turmeric
¼ teaspoon ground white pepper
finely grated zest of 1 lime

1 If using shrimp paste, wrap it in foil and roast in a preheated 180°C oven for 10 minutes.

2 Pound the shrimp paste and the remaining ingredients, along with a pinch of salt, in a mortar and pestle or blend in a food processor until a thick paste forms (if using a food processor, you may need to stop a few times and scrape down the side of the bowl). Refrigerate or freeze until ready to use.

**Tip:** For red curry paste, use 2–3 tablespoons chopped red chillies, or to taste, instead of green. For a yellow or mild curry paste, reduce the chilli to 1–2 tablespoons.

# Harissa

**MAKES ABOUT ¾ CUP (200 G)**
PREP **10 mins** COOK **10 mins, plus resting time**

Harissa is a pungent Moroccan spice paste, made here with roast capsicum. It is often quite fiery, so use with caution!

2 red capsicums (peppers), trimmed,
   seeded and quartered
4–6 small red chillies, seeded and chopped
1½ teaspoons ground cumin
1 teaspoon ground caraway or coriander seeds
2 cloves garlic, very finely chopped

1 Preheat the oven grill to high.

2 Place the capsicum, skin-side up, under the grill in a single layer and cook for 8–10 minutes until the skin blackens and blisters. Transfer to a bowl, cover with plastic wrap and leave for 10 minutes to steam, then peel away the skin and discard, setting the flesh aside.

3 Transfer the roast capsicum flesh to a blender, add the remaining ingredients and blend until smooth. Season with salt and pepper to taste, and refrigerate or freeze until ready to use.

# French dressing

SERVES 4  PREP **5 mins**

**A classic all-rounder, French dressing just loves bitter leaves, tomato and cucumber.**

1 tablespoon extra virgin olive oil
2–3 tablespoons white wine vinegar
2–3 teaspoons Dijon mustard
pinch caster sugar

1 Place all the ingredients in a screw-top jar, secure the lid and shake until combined. Season to taste with salt and pepper.

# Herb dressing

SERVES 4  PREP **5 mins**

**A dressing for delicate salads of chicken or fish.**

1 tablespoon extra virgin olive oil
2–3 tablespoons white balsamic vinegar
2 teaspoons wholegrain mustard
1–2 tablespoons lemon juice
3 tablespoons finely chopped mixed herbs
   such as flat-leaf parsley, chives and mint

1 Place all the ingredients in a screw-top jar, secure the lid and shake until combined. Season to taste with salt and pepper.

# Nam jim dressing

SERVES 4  PREP **5 mins**

**A spicy and tart Asian-style dressing that contains no oil.**

1–2 small red chillies, or to taste, seeded
   and finely chopped
1 clove garlic, crushed
2 teaspoons palm or brown sugar
1–2 tablespoons fish sauce
3 tablespoons lime juice

1 Place all the ingredients in a screw-top jar, secure the lid and shake until combined. Add 1–2 teaspoons water to loosen the dressing if needed, then season to taste with salt and pepper.

# Paprika and honey dressing

SERVES 4  PREP **5 mins**

**A sweet and slightly spicy dressing to be used with salads of lamb, chicken or pork.**

1 tablespoon extra virgin olive oil
2–3 tablespoons sherry vinegar or red wine vinegar
2 teaspoons honey
¼ teaspoon sweet paprika
1 teaspoon seeded mustard

1 Place all the ingredients in a screw-top jar, secure the lid and shake until combined. Season to taste with salt and pepper.

# Garlic yoghurt dressing

SERVES 4  PREP **5 mins**

**A creamy and tangy 'no fat' dressing that goes with just about any type of salad.**

4 tablespoons reduced-fat plain yoghurt
1 clove garlic, crushed
2 tablespoons apple cider vinegar
2 teaspoons Dijon mustard

1 Stir all the ingredients together until well combined. Season to taste with salt and pepper.

# Salad cream

SERVES 6  PREP **5 mins**

**Use this dressing for coleslaw, potato salad or caesar salad, or wherever you want a creamy dressing that's low in fat.**

4 tablespoons reduced-fat mayonnaise
2 tablespoons lemon juice
3 teaspoons horseradish cream
pinch caster sugar

1 Stir all the ingredients together until well combined. Add 1–2 teaspoons water to loosen the dressing if needed, then season to taste with salt and pepper.

# Salsa verde

SERVES 4  PREP **10 mins**

**The strong flavours in this version of the classic green sauce team well with red meat and roast vegetables.**

1 tablespoon extra virgin olive oil
2 anchovy fillets, drained of oil and finely chopped
1 tablespoon finely chopped drained capers
finely grated zest and juice of 1 lemon
2 tablespoons orange juice
1–2 cloves garlic, crushed
3 tablespoons chopped mixed herbs such as flat-leaf
   parsley, mint, chives and basil

1 Blend or pound all the ingredients together until smooth. Add more lemon or orange juice if needed to balance the flavours, then season with salt and pepper to taste.

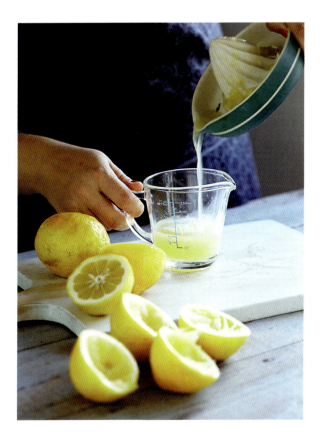

**1 SERVE (1 TABLESPOON) =**
1 unit fat

# Dukkah

MAKES 45 G

PREP **5 mins**  COOK **10 mins**

This is a Middle Eastern spice blend typically scattered over finished dishes for a burst of flavour. It will keep for up to 2 weeks in the fridge.

30 g hazelnuts or blanched almonds
4 tablespoons sesame seeds
2 tablespoons ground coriander
1½ tablespoons ground cumin
pinch cayenne pepper (optional)

1 Preheat the oven to 180°C. Spread the nuts and seeds on a baking tray and roast for 8–10 minutes until golden. If using hazelnuts, wrap them in a tea towel and rub off the skins. Chop the nuts very finely and set aside to cool.

2 Mix all the ingredients together and store in an airtight container.

# Madras curry powder

MAKES 5¼ TABLESPOONS

PREP **5 mins**

This is a mild curry powder. If you like, add a large pinch of cayenne pepper to the mix for a spicier blend.

2 tablespoons ground coriander
1 tablespoon ground cumin
2 teaspoons ground fennel
2 teaspoons ground turmeric
2 teaspoons brown mustard seeds, ground
¼ teaspoon ground cloves
1 teaspoon freshly ground black pepper

1 Mix all the ingredients together and store in an airtight container.

# Cajun spice mix

MAKES 1¾ TABLESPOONS

PREP **5 mins**

Use this to flavour braises or stews, or mix with 2 teaspoons olive oil and use as a marinade for chicken.

2 teaspoons sweet paprika
1 teaspoon ground cumin
1 teaspoon onion powder
1 teaspoon garlic powder
½ teaspoon dried oregano
½ teaspoon dried thyme
¼ teaspoon cayenne pepper

1 Mix all the ingredients together and store in an airtight container.

# Garam masala

MAKES 3¾ TABLESPOONS

PREP **5 mins**

This Indian spice blend is often added to a dish towards the end of the cooking time to add extra flavour.

1 tablespoon ground cumin
1 tablespoon ground coriander
2 teaspoons freshly ground black pepper
2 teaspoons ground cardamom
1 teaspoon ground cinnamon
½ teaspoon ground nutmeg
¼ teaspoon ground cloves

1 Mix all the ingredients together and store in an airtight container.

# Vegetable stock

MAKES ABOUT 2 LITRES
PREP **10 mins** COOK **3 hours 15 mins**

Using a homemade stock is very cost-effective and will make a huge difference to the flavour of soups and stews. The addition of tomatoes, garlic and mushrooms helps to bump up the flavour and give the stock an earthy note. This stock will keep in the fridge for 2–3 days, or you can freeze it in 2 cup (500 ml) portions for up to 2 months.

1 tablespoon vegetable oil
1 onion, chopped
1 leek, white part only, washed and chopped
1 carrot, thickly sliced
2 sticks celery, chopped
140 g button mushrooms, chopped
1 tomato, quartered
4 cloves garlic, chopped
1 strip lemon zest, removed with a vegetable peeler
4 stalks flat-leaf parsley
2 large sprigs thyme
1 bay leaf
8 black peppercorns
1 teaspoon salt

1 Place a large stockpot over medium heat. Add the oil, onion, leek, carrot, celery and mushroom and cook for 10–15 minutes, stirring frequently, until the vegetables are soft. Add the remaining ingredients, along with 3.5 litres water and bring to a very gentle simmer. Skim the surface to remove any impurities, then simmer the stock gently for 2½–3 hours.

2 Strain the stock through muslin or a fine-meshed sieve and leave to cool.

# Chicken stock

MAKES ABOUT 2 LITRES
PREP **10 mins** COOK **3 hours**

Using a variety of chicken pieces to make stock gives a more intense flavour. This stock will keep in the fridge for 2–3 days, or you can freeze it in 2 cup (500 ml) portions for up to 2 months.

1 kg chicken pieces, such as carcasses, necks and wings
1 onion, chopped
1 leek, white part only, washed and chopped
1 carrot, thickly sliced
2 sticks celery, chopped
100 g button mushrooms, chopped
1 strip lemon zest, removed with a vegetable peeler
4 stalks flat-leaf parsley
2 large sprigs thyme
1 bay leaf
8 black peppercorns

1 Place the chicken pieces in a large stockpot and cover generously with cold water. Bring to simmering point and simmer for 5 minutes, skimming the surface to remove any impurities. Add the remaining ingredients, then reduce the heat to maintain a very gentle simmer and cook for 3 hours, skimming the surface from time to time.

2 Strain the stock through muslin or a fine-meshed sieve and leave to cool. Skim any fat from the surface before using.

**Tip:** For a stronger flavoured stock, simmer the strained stock over medium heat until reduced and the desired flavour is achieved. Alternatively, you could roast the chicken bones in a preheated 180°C oven for 25 minutes until browned before adding them to the water – this will give a darker, richer stock.

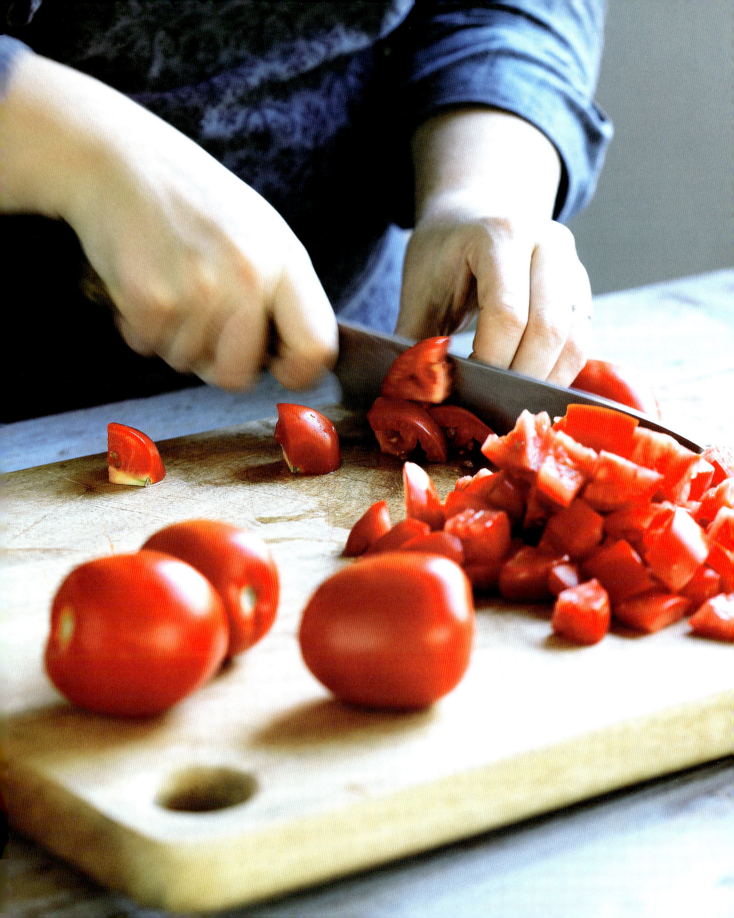

# index

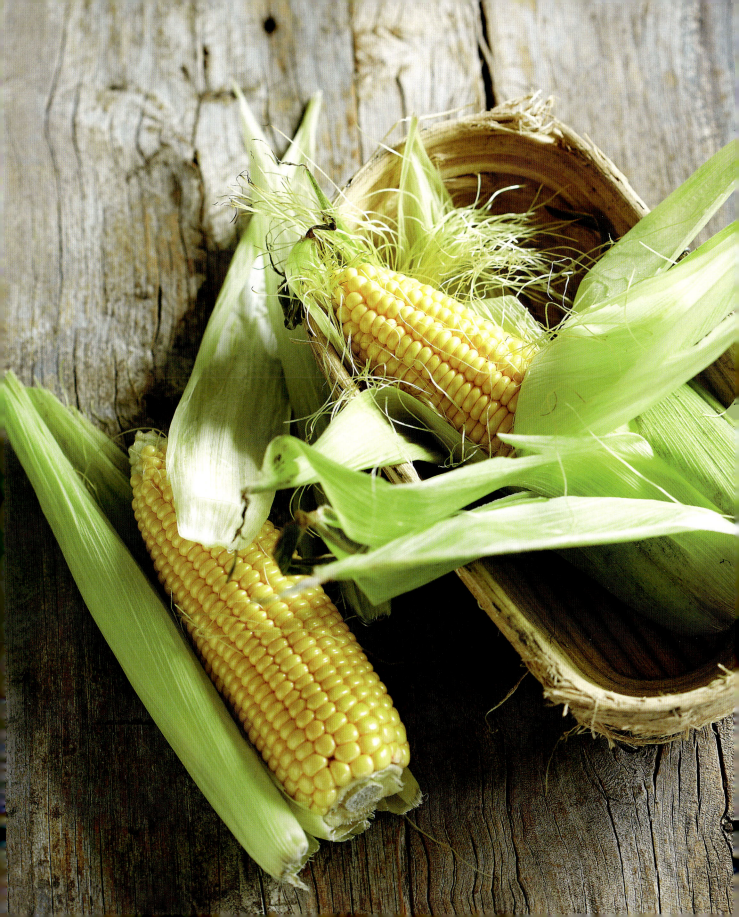

PENGUIN BOOKS

Published by the Penguin Group
Penguin Group (Australia)
707 Collins Street, Melbourne, Victoria 3008, Australia
(a division of Pearson Australia Group Pty Ltd)
Penguin Group (USA) Inc.
375 Hudson Street, New York, New York 10014, USA
Penguin Group (Canada)
90 Eglinton Avenue East, Suite 700, Toronto, Canada ON M4P 2Y3
(a division of Pearson Penguin Canada Inc.)
Penguin Books Ltd
80 Strand, London WC2R 0RL England
Penguin Ireland
25 St Stephen's Green, Dublin 2, Ireland
(a division of Penguin Books Ltd)
Penguin Books India Pvt Ltd
11 Community Centre, Panchsheel Park, New Delhi – 110 017, India
Penguin Group (NZ)
67 Apollo Drive, Rosedale, Auckland 0632, New Zealand
(a division of Pearson New Zealand Ltd)
Penguin Books (South Africa) (Pty) Ltd, Rosebank Office Park, Block D,
181 Jan Smuts Avenue, Parktown North, Johannesburg, 2196, South Africa
Penguin (Beijing) Ltd
7F, Tower B, Jiaming Center, 27 East Third Ring Road North,
Chaoyang District, Beijing 100020, China

Penguin Books Ltd, Registered Offices: 80 Strand, London, WC2R 0RL,
England

First published by Penguin Group (Australia), 2013

10 9 8 7 6 5 4 3 2 1

Introductory text pages 1–7 copyright © CSIRO 2013
Text copyright © Penguin Group (Australia) 2013
Photographs copyright © Cath Muscat 2013

The moral right of the author has been asserted.

Styling by Sarah O'Brien
Recipes by Brett Sargent
Design by Arielle Gamble © Penguin Group (Australia)
Typeset in Minion 11.5/15pt and Din 10.25/14.5pt by Samantha Jayaweera
© Penguin Group (Australia)
Colour separation by Splitting Image Colour Studio, Clayton, Victoria
Printed and bound in China by South China Printing Company

National Library of Australia Cataloguing-in-Publication data:

The CSIRO total wellbeing diet recipes on a budget / CSIRO
9780670076321 (pbk.)
Includes index.
Weight loss. Reducing diets—Recipes. Low budget cooking.
Other authors/contributors: CSIRO.

613.25

penguin.com.au

ACKNOWLEDGEMENTS

The CSIRO acknowledges Professor Manny Noakes, Professor Peter
Clifton, Associate Professor Grant Brinkworth and Belinda Wyld for their
contributions to the CSIRO Total Wellbeing Diet and Exercise program,
as well as Atul Kacker, Pennie Taylor and Andreas Kahl for their work
on this book. Professor Manny Noakes and Associate Professor Grant
Brinkworth also need to be acknowledged for their ongoing research
commitment into the CSIRO Total Wellbeing Diet and Exercise Program.

The organisation also acknowledges Professor Martin Cole for his
ongoing support for this research, and thanks all those who have
funded the research involved in developing the program: CSIRO Animal,
Food and Health Sciences; CSIRO Preventative Health Flagship; Dairy
Australia; Goodman Fielder; Meat and Livestock Australia; the National
Heart Foundation; the National Centre of Excellence in Functional Foods;
the Pork CRC; the Egg Nutrition Council; the Dairy Health and Nutrition
Consortium and the National Health and Medical Research Council.

Thanks to the team at Penguin involved in producing this book:
Julie Gibbs, Katrina O'Brien, Virginia Birch, Arielle Gamble,
Samantha Jayaweera and Elena Cementon. Thanks also to
recipe writer Brett Sargent and the photographic team,
Cath Muscat, Sarah O'Brien and Tina Asher.